REFLECTIVE PRACTICE IN NURSING

The Growth of the Professional Practitioner

Other books of interest

Becoming a Reflective Practitioner
*A reflective and holistic approach to clinical nursing, practice
development and clinical supervision*
Chris Johns
0-632-05561-8

Mentoring, Preceptorship and Clinical Supervision
A Guide to Professional Support Roles in Clinical Practice
Second Edition
Alison Morton-Cooper and Anne Palmer
0-632-04967-7

Successful Supervision in Health Care Practice
Promoting Professional Development
Edited by Jenny Spouse and Liz Redfern
0-632-05159-9

REFLECTIVE PRACTICE IN NURSING

The Growth of the Professional Practitioner

SECOND EDITION

Edited by

SARAH BURNS

BA, RGN, RNT, SCM, DN (Lond)
VSO (Voluntary Services Overseas) Health Trainer,
Savannakhet Provincial Health Services, Lao PDR, SE Asia.

and

CHRIS BULMAN

MSc, BSc. (Hons), RGN, RNT, PGCEA
Senior Lecturer in Nursing and Health Care
School of Health Care, Oxford Brookes University

Blackwell
Science

Blackwell Science Ltd
Editorial Offices:
Osney Mead, Oxford OX2 0EL
25 John Street, London WC1N 2BS
23 Ainslie Place, Edinburgh EH3 6AJ
350 Main Street, Malden
  MA 02148 5018, USA
54 University Street, Carlton
  Victoria 3053, Australia
10, rue Casimir Delavigne
  75006 Paris, France

Other Editorial Offices:

Blackwell Wissenschafts-Verlag GmbH
Kurfürstendamm 57
10707 Berlin, Germany

Blackwell Science KK
MG Kodenmacho Building
7–10 Kodenmacho Nihombashi
Chuo-ku, Tokyo 104, Japan

The right of the Author to be identified as the Author of this Work has been asserted in accordance with the Copyright, Designs and Patents Act 1988.

First edition published 1994
Reprinted 1994, 1995 (twice), 1996 (twice), 1997
Second edition published 2000
Reprinted 2001

Set in 10/12.5 pt Century Book
by DP Photosetting, Aylesbury, Bucks
Printed and bound in Great Britain by
MPG Books Ltd, Bodmin, Cornwall

The Blackwell Science logo is a trade mark of Blackwell Science Ltd, registered at the United Kingdom Trade Marks Registry

DISTRIBUTORS

Marston Book Services Ltd
PO Box 269
Abingdon
Oxon OX14 4YN
(*Orders:* Tel: 01235 465500
        Fax: 01235 465555)

USA
Blackwell Science, Inc.
Commerce Place
350 Main Street
Malden, MA 02148 5018
(*Orders:* Tel: 800 759 6102
                781 388 8250
        Fax: 781 388 8255)

Canada
Login Brothers Book Company
324 Saulteaux Crescent
Winnipeg, Manitoba R3J 3T2
(*Orders:* Tel: 204 837-2987
        Fax: 204 837-3116)

Australia
Blackwell Science Pty Ltd
54 University Street
Carlton, Victoria 3053
(*Orders:* Tel: 03 9347 0300
        Fax: 03 9347 5001)

A catalogue record for this title is available from the British Library

ISBN 0-632-05291-0

Library of Congress
Cataloging-in-Publication Data

Reflective practice in nursing: the growth of the professional practitioner/edited by Sarah Burns and Chris Bulman.—2nd ed.
      p. ; cm.
   Includes bibliographical references and index.
   ISBN 0-632-05291-0 (pbk.)
   1. Nursing—Study and teaching.
2. Nursing—Philosophy. 3. Self-evaluation. 4. Self-knowledge, Theory of. I. Burns, Sarah, DN. II. Bulman, Chris.
   [DNLM: 1. Nursing. 2. Education, Nursing. 3. Learning. 4. Nursing Process. 5. Philosophy, Nursing. 6. Thinking. WY 16 R332 2000]
RT73.R346 2000
610.73'01—dc21   99-088088

For further information on
Blackwell Science, visit our website:
www.blackwell-science.com

*This book is dedicated
to the late Donald Schön
whose work has been such
an inspiration to us*

Contents

List of Contributors

Sue Atkins, *MSC, RN, RM, Dip N, DipN Ed*, Principal Lecturer in Nursing and Health Care, School of Health Care, Oxford Brookes University.

Ysanne Chapman, *RN, BEd (Nursing), MSc Hons, DNE, GDE*, PhD Scholar, Department of Clinical Nursing, University of Adelaide.

Nettie Dearmun, *PhD, BSc (Hons), RGN, RCSN, DN (Lond), DNE, RNT, ITEC*, Principal Lecturer, Oxford Brookes University; Field Chair for Children's Nursing and Senior Nurse, Oxford Radcliffe Trust.

Cath Davies, *RGN, RNT, MSc, BSc (Hons)*, formerly Lecturer-Practitioner, School of Health Care, Oxford Brookes University and Oxford Radcliffe Trust.

Sue Duke, *MSc, BSc (Hons), RGN, RNT, ONC, PG Dip*, Lecturer-Practitioner, School of Health Care, Oxford Brookes University and Sir Michael Sobell House, Oxford.

Mary FitzGerald, *RN, DipN, Cert Ed, MN, PhD*, Senior Lecturer, Department of Clinical Nursing, University of Adelaide.

Bev Gillings, *BSc (Hons), PGCE, MSc, RGN, RNT*, Senior Lecturer in Nursing and Health Care, Oxford Brookes University.

Brigid Reid, *RGN, BN (Hons), Cert Ed, MPhil*, Head of Nursing (Surgery), Heartland's and Solihull NHS Trust (Teaching).

Pam Sharp, *PGDip (Ed), PGDip (Advanced Health Care Practice)*, Senior Lecturer in Nursing and Health Care, School of Health Care, Oxford Brookes University.

Preface

Reflective practice: '... a process of reviewing an experience of practice in order to describe, analyse and evaluate and so inform learning from practice'.

(Reid 1993, p. 305)

Welcome to the second edition of *Reflective Practice in Nursing*. In keeping with the definition of reflection above, this is a book about learning from experience. Since the publication of the first edition of this book, reflection has become a key word within nursing education, and judging by the amount of debate and investigation in the literature it is a concept that has got 'under the skins' of practitioners.

This new edition responds to the interest among nurses in mastering the fundamental skills of reflective practice. It offers a motivating and accessible text that documents and analyses the increase in knowledge and skills related to reflection that have been developing over the past five years. We hope it will provide a route to communicate our growing knowledge and expertise about reflective practice, which originated in Oxfordshire as a result of an approach to nurse education that values and supports the development of reflective practice. This book does not assume any previous knowledge about reflection and aims to provide a text of practical use for those wanting to learn about reflection and what it may have to offer them. It remains essentially a book to 'dip' into so that the reader can seek out particular areas of interest according to their own needs rather than feel an obligation to read the whole book from cover to cover.

The first edition of *Reflective Practice in Nursing* has been read by a wide variety of nurses from pre- and post-registration students, to diploma and master's level. It has appealed to practitioners from a huge range of backgrounds and experience, as well as to teachers, managers and mentors. Although research in reflective practice still needs to be done, (indeed this is something on our agenda for the near future) our own continuing work and experience with reflective practice keeps us committed to a process which has the potential to help nurses to learn from their practice.

The second edition includes some exciting and interesting work on developing 'building blocks' for reflection: self awareness, description, analysis, synthesis and evaluation. There are also many new exemplars to allow you to share in the work of other reflective practitioners at all levels of expertise. In Oxford we continue to grade students on their ability to reflect on their experiences in practice but we have been challenged to develop new ways to do this. Therefore you will also find plenty to challenge your thinking regarding the assessment of reflection in today's nursing climate, as well as ideas and suggestions for assessing reflective practice. This will be of particular interest to teachers and students.

A practical examination of reflection and clinical supervision is included, which we hope will prove a real help to practitioners and managers trying to develop their practice through clinical supervision. There is some new research work on mentoring and the competency development of students using reflective practice and on qualified nurses who have had a reflective pre-registration education. We feel there is much inspiration to be gathered from the chapters exploring the experiences of students and of the experienced practitioner in developing reflective practice. In fact as you will see there are two chapters which address the differing concerns of students since we see this as a vital area to explore in relation to reflective practice and its utilisation in nursing. There is also an updated chapter on the theories of reflection for learning.

We hope this book will be helpful to all those involved and interested in developing, using and investigating reflective nursing.

Chris Bulman and Sarah Burns

References

Reid, B. (1993) 'But we're doing it already!' Exploring a response to the concept of reflective practice in order to improve its facilitation. *Nurse Education Today*, **13** 305–9.

Chapter 1
Theories of Reflection for Learning

Introduction

This chapter appears at the beginning of the book but does not necessarily imply that theories should be studied before practice. While intellectual ruminations are interesting and may be helpful, an appreciation of these views is not essential to the nursing student who wants to learn from reflection. Indeed, most of the readers of this chapter will have learnt from their reflections on experience without studying the literature referred to here, and they will almost certainly find their experience useful when considering the following examination of the subject. On the other hand an intellectual enquiry concerning reflection in nursing is necessary for those who recommend, and in some instances dictate, its use.

Despite a number of warnings in the literature to be careful before the wholesale application of critical reflection as a learning tool, critical reflection is favoured and accepted as a dominant discourse in many schools of nursing. The amount of nursing literature in the area has continued to grow but the majority of this literature, with some exceptions, is descriptive and there is little evaluation of the method as a means of learning to nurse. Well thought out and presented theoretical papers do contribute to the debate, however there is a need for research that provides evidence regarding the effectiveness of the technique in nursing (Greenwood 1993, Burnard 1995, Clark, James & Kelly 1996, Clinton 1998).

Turner (1990) and Shapiro (1991) both recommend scepticism in relation to 'grand discourses', that is dominant ideas. Two reasons for this caution are that one prevalent discussion simply replaces another; and that the notions associated with the dominant discourse become so influential that alternative views, especially those of the minority, are likely to be marginalised. While there is a need to be wary of grand discourses, the ideas of learning from reflection on and in *action or* experience (Schön, 1987) are attractive to nurses not least because the approach focuses upon practice and values experience. Nursing writers agree with Adler (1991) that the time to review critically what we mean by learning through reflection or the reflective practitioner is more than ripe. In order that this potentially useful perspective can be appreciated in a temperate fashion we would reiterate that there also is a need to investigate the effect this type of learning has on nurses, both during and after their training. (See the research work of Brigid Reid and Nettie Dearmun within this book.)

In this chapter we review different views of reflection for learning, concentrating on two in particular. Following this we consider the process of reflective learning, although we are cautious here because from our own lonely experiences in the early days of reflecting critically on our nursing practice, and from the frustrated pleas of students for direction, we know that people turn hopefully to the literature for some 'how to' directions. It seems that there is no recipe for how to 'do reflection' but there are plenty of issues worth considering. We believe that the reader will find the other chapters in the book more useful; their descriptions of the experience of learning through reflection may seem more realistically and practically accessible, particularly in view of the years of experience the authors now have in using critical reflection on and in nursing practice. Penultimately there is a discussion of the continuing attraction that this way of learning has for contemporary nurses, including some notes of caution. Lastly there is a discussion of research and reflection.

Views of reflection for learning

Reflection on and in action and critical enquiry have been chosen for most attention, because they are the perspectives referred to most often when nurses discuss learning through critical reflection. They were the ones studied and referred to when the Oxford nursing curriulum was created and established (George (1986), Oxford Brookes University (1988), Champion (1992)).

Of course there are other theoretical views of reflection and these should be acknowledged as legitimate, even if they are not particularly suited to the way we wish to learn the craft of nursing. For instance Descartes (1984, p.127), the modern proponent of reductionism, exemplified by the infamous mind–body split, immortalised the idea of the power of thought in his maxim 'I am thinking therefore I exist'. As a significant figure in the development of modern empirical science his notion of learning through reflection is not what most of the current nursing educationalists have in mind when they refer to 'the reflective practitioner'. In a literature search Adler (1991, p.139) found several different meanings ascribed to reflection and she argued that there is a pressing need for clarification of perspective to avoid quite understandable confusion.

For instance Benner (1984) and Benner & Wrubel (1989) in their endeavour to uncover the concepts of expert nursing and caring ask nurses to reflect and recount their experiences. However their main focus, quite legitimately as phenomenologists, is upon discovering the essence of the phenomenon rather than the narrator's formal learning. It may be that the recounting of the experience leads the narrator to new understandings and that educationalists may use the work in this manner. However, in this instance, phenomenology is a research methodology not a learning technique. Learning from reflection involves students critically analysing and interpreting their own work, albeit with help in some cases from a mentor, preceptor or coach.

Reflection is an idea used in ordinary and educational life. On the one hand reflection is a loosely used concept, easily assimilated into spontaneous everyday action, and on the other hand it can become a complex, difficult to explain and perplexing phenomenon. The straightforward definition of the verb, to reflect, is 'to cast back (light, heat, etc.), to give back or show an image of; to think carefully, meditate on'. (*The Macquarie Dictionary*, 1991.) However philosophical enquiry regarding the nature of human knowledge (epistemology) leads the investigator to alternative and more elaborate conceptions of the process of acquiring knowledge from reflection.

A grasp of the epistemological perspective taken personally, collectively as a profession or adopted by others is revelatory because these perspectives show how knowledge is sought, developed, appreciated and indeed why one view of knowledge might deviate from another view (Sater 1988, Robinson & Vaughan 1992). People's way of pursuing truth affects why and how they reflect, what the outcomes of the process of reflection might be and the language they use to portray it. For example the person who believes in an absolute truth pursued through deductive reasoning will reflect in a logical analytical way in order to make a correct decision and defend the decision using words like 'reliability' and 'generalisability'. This logical deductive reasoning is a form of reflection we appreciate as a perspective held to be useful by many, although one which some may argue is limited by its nature.

In the field of nursing Clarke (1986) wrote one of the earliest papers describing the use of reflection for professional development and based it on John Shotter's theories of the psychology of personal action. Clarke (1986, p.5) mentions that Shotter aimed to conform to the scientific paradigm. I would suggest that this approach is perceptible in a much later paper by a colleague of Clarke's, Newell (1992, p.1327) who proffers the argument that·

'The issues of bias in forgetting and selection at acquisition suggest that accurate reflection may be either impossible or so fundamentally flawed as to be of little value.'

In the paper Newell uses the language of empirical science and the methods of behavioural psychologists to criticise and solve problems he sees in work that originates from a different epistemological perspective. This other perspective, Schön (1987) argues, acknowledges and accepts uncertainty and subjective experience as valid. Appreciation of Schön's approach is essential to a critique of his work. From a similar perspective to Newell, Clinton (1998) gives another astute critique of reflection in action, seriously questioning its value as a learning method for nursing.

The understanding that philosophical circumspection can bring to a subject is the reason why a number of the authors, when considering reflection as a learning method, give an epistemological preamble to their work: Mezirow (1981), Schön (1983) and (1987), Carr & Kemmis (1986), Smyth (1986), and Street (1988). It is necessary in a critique of the literature surrounding reflection to appraise the perspective the author/s are coming from.

Reflection on and in action

Learning by thinking on experience is not a new concept; Dewey (1933) is usually acknowledged as the first educationalist to write about reflection on experience. Nurses became intrigued by the subject as nursing education in the tertiary sector was developed (Deakin University 1988, Oxford Brookes University 1988). There is a particular interest in the work of Schön (1983 and 1987) who describes learning for professional work. Schön devotes considerable space in both books to epistemological arguments regarding the inappropriate dominance of technical rationality in professional education. He describes technical rationality as:

'an epistemology of practice derived from positivist philosophy, built into the very foundations of the modern research university. Technical rationality holds that practitioners are instrumental problem solvers who select technical means best suited to particular purposes. Rigorous professional practitioners solve well-informed instrumental problems by applying theory and technique derived from systematic preferably scientific knowledge.

(Schön 1987, pp.3–4)

This positivistic stance is suited to solving simple problems in contrived situations, rather than the complex, urgent and often surprising problems Schön knows practitioners deal with in practice. Furthermore, people taking the technical rational view do not give credit to the practitioners' demonstrated intellectual agility in practice. Schön (1983 and 1987) posits that knowledge is embedded in and demonstrated through the artistry of everyday practice, in clever things done 'on the job' and yet which are typically so difficult to describe linguistically and, to the frustration of positivistic scientists, impossible to control.

Argyris & Schön (1974, 1978) have developed the idea of 'theory in use'. They propose that practitioners choose their actions with due consideration for the particular situation and use theories generated from their repertoire which is made up of experience, education, values, beliefs and past strategies. Often these theories are implicit in spontaneous behaviour and surface only upon reflection on performance, or when the person is confronted with a problem in practice and has to think deliberately which course of action to take.

Reflection in action is the process whereby the practitioner recognises a new situation or a problem and thinks about it while still acting. Schön (1987) and Boud & Walker (1991) believe it is possible to encourage reflection in action and improve the practitioner's ability to identify problems in the social milieu (enframe problems) and attend to the relevant surrounding stimuli in order to deal with these problems immediately. While problems are not usually exactly the same as on previous occasions, the skilled practitioner is able to select, remix or recast responses from previous experiences, when deciding how to solve a problem in practice. It should be noted that knowledge of conventional theories may be part of the practitioner's repertoire and play a part in the reflection in action. Clinton (1998, p.201) has most reservations about reflection in action as critical reflection. He states;

> 'reflection in action is not reflective in the sense of being an hermeneutic that can be reassessed. It does not involve second or still higher order accounts of nursing practice and does not involve reflexivity. Moreover, it is impossible to derive from it any link between the actions of nurses and reasons for them that may be grounded in a major premise. Consequently, reflection in action leaves nurses bereft of grounds for supposing that the awareness that accompanies practice is reflective in any reflexive sense.'

Reflection on action on the other hand is the retrospective contemplation of practice undertaken in order to uncover the knowledge used in a particular situation, by analysing and interpreting the information recalled. The reflective practitioner may speculate how the situation might have been handled differently and what other knowledge would have been helpful.

This reflective process is far more flexible and realistic than the technical rational approach in which espoused theories, those talked about and taught away from the practice arena, are expected, but cannot hope, to accommodate all of the complications that arise in practical situations. These espoused theories are rejected by some practitioners because in the social world there are hectic variables that are impossible to control. Contextual problems require solutions geared to the precise situation rather than solutions that are general and context free. We would suggest there are few more hectic areas of practice than those encountered by nurses and so aptly described by Cox & Moss (1988) in their paper entitled 'Promiscuous knowledge: the chaos of practice'. Schön's ability to appreciate this working world is a reason why his exposition on professional learning is so welcome to nurses.

Precise theories of safe drug administration are an example of espoused theories taught in class. In practice, however, a nurse may well decide, in the patient's best interest, to deviate in some way from the protocol. Some might counter that this example simply demonstrates that espoused theories in the real world should be used in a dis-criminatory way, as indeed Benner (1984) found expert nurses do. We would argue that it is this practical ability nurses have to use various sources of knowledge in a flexible way which is so impressive. This ability to discriminate 'on the job' is a clue to proficient and productive nursing, so eminently worth studying and encouraging through reflec-tion on and in action.

That is not to say that espoused theories are to be thrown out with the bath water. Abstract and general theories are needed to inform nurses. The point is that nurses weigh up each problem as it arises and come to a decision in the light of espoused knowledge and the particulars of the situation.

Critical enquiry

Philosophically critical enquiry predominantly stems from the work of Habermas and other members of the Frankfurt School, although Carr & Kemmis (1986, p. 32) refer as far back as Aristotle when making their epistemological introduction to critical enquiry. Accordingly Carr & Kemmis (1986, pp. 33–4) support Aristotle's notion that the appro-priateness of knowledge acquisition depends on the purpose that it serves. Habermas (1977), in a similar vein describes three areas of human interest from which knowledge may arise. These areas are *technical* interests that result in instrumental work guided by empirical knowledge; *practical* interests which are concerned with communication and intersubjectivity, guided by knowledge that provides understanding; and, lastly, *emancipatory* interests which are concerned with social equity, freedom and justice guided by knowledge discovered through a process of 'conscientisation'. Freire (1972) explains conscientisation as a dawning awareness, of competing human interests and power structures that, in effect, manufacture and perpetuate social situations. Mezirow (1981, p. 5) explains that the latter domain is termed emancipatory because it leads people to a true understanding of the cause of their predicaments and hopefully a pathway to their resolution of them.

Relating emancipatory interests to nursing (as Carr & Kemmis (1986, p. 32) have related this domain to teaching), nurses develop competence through a process of critical reflection on experience, they examine their work and the contribution their nursing, and nursing generally, makes socially. Then in turn they also consider the effect social forces have upon themselves and their work. The notion of informed action or praxis is an important concept to critical theorists, one that is developed through the reciprocal relationship between action and critical reflection. The resulting heightened awareness and the revelation of the variety of factors that contribute to an established order can be used deliberately by people to understand, and in some instances rearrange, the social order in which they find themselves, in the name of justice and freedom.

By emancipation critical theorists refer to the freedom gained by people to contribute in a legitimate way to social systems that are equitable and just. The power to contribute equitably is achieved by those who learn how a situation is established and perpetuated. Emancipatory knowledge is gained from a broad perspective whereby issues are considered that are beyond the immediate situation, such as the historical and political elements of the situation. Critical reflection involves Schön's (1987, p. 93) notion of the student *extraordinarily re-experiencing the ordinary*. This fresh view of everyday experience renders problematic things such as previously accepted value and belief systems and routines, generating questions such as how are these ordinary things connected to economic, political and social exigencies? This new thinking can reveal distortions, that is those contributions, from unexpected sources, to the maintenance of the status quo. For instance students may come to appreciate their own contribution to a situation in which they are oppressed. Freire (1972, p. 376) suggests this type of knowledge ('conscientisation') equips people with the information needed to change situations radically, rather than to make superficial cosmetic alterations which serve in the long term to perpetuate injustice and allow current power relationships to persist. The idea of distortions is a particularly important one. It is quite possible that students reflecting critically on their own may not have the resources to see the distortions that they bring to their perspective and can exaggerate through the process of reflection. This is a particular strength of the reflective supervision described by Johns (1994a) and Johns & Freshwater (1998).

Freire (1972) wrote of social revolution that would free both oppressors and the oppressed, but he warned against the possibility of the oppressed mimicking the behaviour of the oppressors, once the former obtained power. For it would then be likely that one oppressive system would replace another, and no lasting improvement would be achieved. While the critical theorists talk of social change, not all believe revolution is inevitable. Critical reflection will attune the student to the motives and perspectives of other parties in the social milieu, and this improved understanding of the situation may demonstrate that other interests, besides one's own, have a legitimate place in a just society.

Other theorists aligned to the critical approach are Marx and Freud. They are defined as critical because of Marx's notions of the critique of ideology (influential connected ideas that legitimise oppression), and because of Freud's psychoanalysis, whereby through self reflection people can rediscover their self and the conditions they are in which may be repressive (Carr & Kemmis 1986, p. 138). These sociological and psychological theories are good examples of how critical enquiry may lead to both personal growth and social improvement.

It is apparent that Schön's widely used work differs from the critical theorists. Schön concentrates predominantly on the development of the individual student's ability to address problems and develop skills in their particular context. He does not challenge the curriculum or call for social change. Adler (1991) notes for instance that Schön is predominantly interested in achieving the goals prescribed by the curriculum, for example learning to do the job efficiently. On the other hand while the critical theorists incorporate a responsibility for the broader social scene in their work, they are criticised for their impracticality. Besides raising consciousness they do not demonstrate how students might bring about change (Bell & Schniedewind 1987).

An approach that incorporates the theories of Schön and the critical enquirers may be possible and may help to re-establish a balanced approach to nursing education in the following two areas. In the wake of the pervasive influence of humanistic ideas in recent times, nursing could be criticised for concentrating too much on the individual, rather than the collective problems of society. Bevis & Watson (1989) talk of the need for nursing education to find a balance between the focus on the individual micro perspective and the social macro perspective. Another balance needed is that between academic freedom, for example the freedom to pursue intellectual pathways that the individual deems appropriate, and the need for nursing students to acquire skills in order to protect the public from incompetent practitioners. These are problems we have to face and try to accommodate.

We are not suggesting that Schön's ideas and the work of critical theorists should be merged, there are too many differences for that. They may be used in a complementary fashion. Schön's techniques for learning practical skills and coaching students enable them to achieve competence in certain prescribed areas necessary to guarantee certain standards of professional work. The critical aspect incorporates a healthily sceptical view (so necessary for critical thinking) of phenomena encountered in the educational process and encourages intellectual consideration of other options. It is a broader perspective that incorporates the students' search for an understanding of the social world and the ways in which this broader context affects them. It is only fair to help students to understand the differences between these two approaches to learning, in order that they can understand their role and objectives in the educational process using reflection for learning.

The pre-registration nursing courses are bound by the regulations of the statutory bodies to achieve certain standards and competencies, which means that some compromises have to be made in terms of the student's freedom to choose experience that is most meaningful to them. We propose that curricula for advanced nursing courses need not be constrained by the need to acquire prescribed skills, and that an emancipatory approach to learning could be adopted without compromise. Perhaps in some of the post-registration courses and course work for Master of Nursing degrees this should be considered. Wheeler & Chinn (1991) describe a feminist and emancipatory style of learning in which the group shares responsibility for devising the learning experience.

The process

The process of reflection for learning is dealt with in the educational literature, particularly explicitly in Schön (1987), Boud, Keogh & Walker (1985) and Boud & Walker (1991). Schön provides examples of students and coaches working together to analyse and learn from experience. Boud, Keogh & Walker (1985) have developed and refined (Boud & Walker, 1991) a model for reflective learning, which incorporates phases of preparation, experience, reflective processes and outcomes. Examples of recent nursing literature which, on the whole, has used the above authors' work and applied it to nursing situations are Emden (1991), Gray & Forsstrom (1991) and Cox, Hickson & Taylor (1991). Atkins and Murphy (1993, p. 1190) reviewed the literature on reflection and identify the skills most likely to be required for the process of reflection for learning. These skills range from self awareness, to the following abilities: describe experiences; critically analyse situations; develop new perspectives and evaluate the learning process. (See Sue Atkins' chapter for further analysis of these skills.) Glen (1995) and Schank (1990) link critical thinking with reflection suggesting that reflection can highlight the 'imaginative speculation' often missing in rational, linear processes such as the nursing process. Suggesting that both personal and professional reflection are necessary steps in the development of a nurse who has personal integrity, (Glen 1995, p. 174) makes a plea to educators to return to the classical values of teaching 'how' to think rather than 'what' to think. Through practising reflection, Glen (1995) and Schank (1990, p. 89) agree that students of nursing will learn a skill that is not only useful in today's health systems, but is essential to enable nurses to rise to challenges and be oriented to the future.

Yet this type of learning is so personal it is doubtful that the literature can offer more than helpful suggestions. One such proposal (Graham 1995) considers the introduction of action learning groups as a suitable method by which students can possibly move from the notions of reflection-*on*-practice towards reflection-*in* practice. Readers will find that the other chapters in this book offer a great deal in terms of descriptions of how reflection for learning is carried out, these accounts provide refreshing examples of unconventional and imaginative innovations. The literature however brings some issues to mind that are worth considering during the process of learning by reflection on experience.

The educationalists write of the potential difficulties that students will have reflecting critically and of the importance of expert support. Nursing students' difficulties are compounded in that they have to contend not only with dawning self awareness, but practice situations in which they encounter a plethora of different emotions ranging from ecstatic relief to despair, fear, suffering, disgust and distress. It is good that nurses are encouraged to surface and examine their reactions to these phenomena through reflection. All too often in the past reactions have been repressed and must have contributed significantly to stress among nurses (Lawler 1991, Smith 1992). However these reactions can be expected and lecturers, mentors and lecturer practitioners need to be prepared to support the students. While post-registered nurses may not feel as stressed in practice because they become familiar with their practice area, they have different stresses related to increasing responsibility at work. Johns describes work done with registered nurses to help them to unravel the mysteries and stresses embedded in their practice.

Johns, in work that has spanned over ten years, examines in detail the work of supervisor and nurses learning through reflection (Johns 1994a, 1994b, 1995, 1996, and Johns and Freshwater 1998). His work has been with post-registered nurses and he typically reports on case studies, using reflection on his own work as a supervisor to generate understanding of the process. He has developed and gradually refined a model of structured reflection that involves intensive and systematic examination and analysis of a particular experience. (See the exemplar chapter at the end of the book and further reference to his work in Chapter 5 by Bev Gillings on clinical supervision.) The learning experience is supervised so that students receive guidance and support through their critical reflections on practice. This type of individual attention is time consuming and probably impractical, in the present economic climate, in large undergraduate schools.

Learning through reflection is a laborious and deliberate process. It does not just occur, nor is it something that is done in one's head on the way home. Thoughts on actions need to be articulated, either verbally or in writing. The work needs to be analysed critically, interpreted and compared with other perspectives. Schön (1987) describes reflective conversations where ideas are shared and debated, Boud, Keogh & Walker (1985) describe debriefing after experience and Holly (1987) details keeping a professional journal. Space for this type of work needs to be built into the learning syllabus. It is hoped that there will come a time when reflection on action will be valued to such an extent that it can be given official time during the working day, when nurses can write about or discuss their experiences with the mutual purpose of learning from them. There is little evidence of the widespread adoption of reflective learning as part of working nurses' daily schedule. Reflection is usually done as part of a unit of study and then only if it is tied to assessment.

Garrison (1991) writes that learning through reflection is a learning technique most suited to adults who have a wealth of past experience and an intellectual maturity to cope with autonomy, differing perspectives and shifting ideas. Even so, in Usher's (1985) experience most students initially find learning from experience strange. They are, on the whole, more comfortable learning facts from books. Richardson (Richardson R., 1995) however, cautions that mechanisation of the process of reflection may reinforce the very thing that reflective practice is trying to negate. By setting up reflection as an 'elitist' function Richardson (1995, p.1049) purports that the theory–practice gap lends itself to be widened, rather than closed. In keeping with other contemporary authors (see Glen (1995) and Schank (1990), for example) Richardson defends reflection as a non-linear process that has the potential to create opportunities for nurses to integrate both art and science aspects of our profession if used in a creative way.

Restricted views of learning and a measure of reluctance to learn through reflection on practice, stem from issues such as past learning methods and traditional attitudes towards learning and education. Usher (1985) examines the issue of authority and suggests that however democratic teachers want to be they do exercise considerable authority and power in the learning situation. The sources of this power are the direction and outcome of the learning and the assessment of the student's progress. When the students do not have autonomy then it is likely that they will look to the teacher for direction and learn what they think the teacher wants them to, rather than what seems most relevant to them. It is, in these cases, frustrating for students to be given little direction.

The problem regarding student autonomy is particularly relevant to nursing where students are given direction because certain competence is required in order to register before practising, and in instances where clinical practice is assessed and graded according to the student's ability to reflect critically upon their experience. (Murphy & Reading 1992, also see Pam Sharp and Cath Davies' chapter on assessment and evaluation of reflection, Chapter 3). When they have to achieve in order to succeed in a course, students can feel insecure and somewhat frustrated when there are no firm directions about what constitutes good reflection and how marks can be obtained. Some direction is given to them in the form of specific competencies they need to master during the course. A measure of freedom may appear when the students are encouraged to reflect critically on their experiences and develop expertise and produce exemplars from their practice. When writing about their professional experiences they choose what examples to use themselves. However it is naive to think that the system is perfect and the degree of control over what nursing students learn is a potential obstruction to radical learning and out of tune with emancipatory pedagogy.

A critical, yet pertinent view of the power relationships emanating from the increasing use of journal writing as a pedagogical strategy is argued as problematic by Wellard and Bethune (1996). They suggest that the process of engaging in reflection is not the panacea towards the making of an 'authentic nurse' Wellard and Bethune (1996, p.1080), and caution that students may be caught between 'a rock and a hard place' when 'journalling' about their practice. Using Foucault's analysis Wellard and Bethune regard students as 'docile' bodies who, in their need to articulate their image of nursing as 'ideal', sometimes ignore the realities of their world of practice. They further argue that relationships between students and others within the clinical setting are tenuous at the best of times, and potentially moderate students' willingness to 'tell it how it is'. From their experience as university lecturers in nursing, while in agreement with the concept of reflection, Wellard and Bethune (1996) identify students' powerlessness as a likely negative outcome, especially in clinical situations where students resist relating their own observations of 'what is' happening. Their silences can be as futile as their 'fictional fantasies' yet these undesired outcomes are perpetuated by underestimating the impact of the powerful relationships between students and lecturers, and/or students and clinicians. Wellard and Bethune do not suggest that we should throw the baby out with the bath water. Rather they propose the employment of strategies that permit a continual questioning of the need for the unqualified use of reflection in nursing courses and a increased consciousness that in clinical practice students may need a modicum of encouragement to give voice to what they see. Reflective journal writing can then live up to some of those promises articulated in the earlier literature and thus succeed in advancing students' practices.

However it is possible that the reverse of Wellard and Bethune's (1996) proposition is true. As mentioned earlier, a really important part of critical theory is the ironing out of distortions. There is the potential for students to exaggerate distortions when relating stories from the field unless they are facilitated by people who are able to draw out other perspectives and include them in the analysis. This is not always possible for lecturers who do not have a good knowledge of the context to which the student relates, or who perhaps lack a sympathy for situations in practice that are less than ideal.

Nursing and reflection on experience

The appeal of reflective learning to the nursing profession has a number of sources, which involve areas such as nursing's history, ideologies and social circumstances. These provide a stronger rationale for the appeal than the rather perjorative explanation given by some that reflective learning is just another fad in nursing.

In order to build a discipline and inform the profession, nurses are trying to find suitable means of knowledge acquisition; ways by which they can acknowledge and accommodate the subjective, unpredictable nature of the world in which they work. For a long time now, nurses have written of a growing sense of the limitations of traditional positivistic science. Schumacher and Gortner (1992) describe contemporary or post-positivistic thinking in the philosophy of science and suggest that arguments against traditional science are somewhat late. Ideas in the philosophy of science are in a state of change and logical positivism is generally considered obsolete (Holmes 1991, Menke 1983, Schumacher & Gortner 1992, FitzGerald 1996). Indeed there has been a trend since the 1960s to dismiss the notions of theory-neutral observations, absolute truth and a static world as realistically impossible. This scepticism was encouraged by the work of the historicists notably Kuhn (1970) and Laudan (1977). While we appreciate this point and believe that nurses have, as Holmes (1991) writes, been somewhat late in assimilating topical philosophical ideas, there is still evidence that traditional views remain dominant in practical spheres. This is especially so in the areas that impinge on the practical world of nurses, for example the style of research accepted by funding bodies and ethics committees; the style of management within the health service (which is still bureaucratic, medically dominated and product-driven); and, relevant to this chapter, education. If nurses are to take new paths towards knowledge acquisition it is important for them to be able to explain and justify the practice discipline of nursing. This will be possible, it is suggested, if we investigate and thoroughly understand nursing practice.

Historically nurse education has been dominated by medical tradition and hence positivistic, reductionist approaches. Evidence of this influence can be seen in old curricula with theory taught (often from other disciplines) and applied to practice. This perspective has contributed to the division of theory and practice (Munhall 1982, Alexander 1983). Theories generated away from practice have been, on the whole unsuccessfully, applied to the practice situation. As Pearson (1992) also suggests, this traditional approach has led to the devaluation of the practice of nursing, as status is given to thinkers rather than doers. These problems have been recognised and deliberated upon by nurses for a long time, and as explained by Miller (1985), the means of overcoming them has been sought in a variety of ways. Cox *et al.* (1991, p. 374) proffer the notion that professional work and disciplinary knowledge are synergistic when, through praxis (thoughtful action), they actively complement one another.

In a concise exposition Schön (1983, 1987) describes the crisis in confidence in professional knowledge (Schön 1983, p. 3). There is a growing mistrust brought about by a suspicion that espoused theories from academia are inadequate for the preparation or continuing development of professional practitioners. There have been, and indeed still are, similar signs of dissatisfaction with nurse education manifest through the following:

- new practitioners who believe that their preparation was inadequate (UKCC 1986);
- the anti-intellectual lobby, 'you don't need degrees to nurse, what's wrong with good old-fashioned caring';
- the frustrated nursing students reading for post-registration certificates and degrees who find their study material divorced from their reality;
- the relatively slow development and appreciation of the discipline of nursing by nurses at all levels in practice institutions.

While it can be argued that all the arguments listed have some flaws, and are at times critical in an irresponsible way, it is reasonable that nurses should wish academics and educationalists to pay attention to their actions. Most nurses wish to have their considerable abilities appreciated and used to contribute to the growing body of knowledge for the discipline of nursing. However this will only be achieved when it is possible to make explicit what it is that nurses do so well. Benner (1984) and Benner & Wrubel (1989) have done a great deal through their phenomenological research to clarify and enhance the value of the art of expert nursing. This type of clarity can be obtained, suggest Perry & Moss (1989), by practitioners who are prepared to examine their work in a critically reflective way. Reflection on action, in writing, conversations and discussions should help nurses to develop the ability to articulate their craft.

Lumby (1991 and 1992) eloquently explains the need for nurses to develop a language of nursing to express the discipline adequately – a language that accommodates an appreciation of the subjective, wonderful and unpredictable nature of the world and which provides a means to justify fair and meaningful ways of sharing and evaluating nursing work. Familiar 'scientific' language has limited nurses by words like 'sample', 'objectivity', 'generalisability' and 'validity'. These words are classically used to justify experimental work and do not suit the interpretive and creative work nurses are generating. What is required is syntax that portrays the exquisite sensitivity of the art and science of nursing and that denotes its unique world. Lumby (1991) exhorts nurses to identify and publicly discuss nursing praxis, exercising, refining and developing our rhetoric, otherwise we may remain constrained in the world of medicine. Reflection on and in action is an essential fuel for such conversations.

Popular and persuasive ideas among nurses are that the practice of nursing is the focus of the discipline (Benner 1984, Watson 1985, Pearson 1988, 1991 and 1992, Gray & Forsstrom 1991) and an important source of knowledge. Cox *et al.* (1991, p. 373) describe nursing as 'careful people-orientated work, which is energised by knowledge', a knowledge that is embedded in the practice of nursing. Attention turned upon nursing work, one example of which is critical reflection on action, is most appropriate for the generation and acquisition of contemporary nursing knowledge.

Courses in the tertiary education sector have resulted in standards which require that nurses are adequately prepared to practise and furthermore to pursue practice in an intellectual way (Oxford Polytechnic, 1988). Critical reflection upon practice appears to be an appropriate approach to combine an appreciation for action and critical enquiry in an academically and practically acceptable way. Although to date there has been little evidence that it is a learning method that endures past formal courses and becomes a part of the life long learning of most professional nurses. (See Nettie Dearmun's chapter, Chapter 8, for exploratory research in this area.)

Emden (1991) contends that a responsible aspiration of all mature nurses is to become a reflective practitioner capable of improving practice by asking difficult questions and being sceptical of practices taken for granted. She describes a process of empowerment and emancipation through critical awareness of an individual's nursing work and situation. Furthermore it is a process which is also useful for members of nursing faculties who continue to develop their practice knowledge as well as their nursing expertise.

Gray & Forsstrom (1991, p. 355) describe a project where they used 'the reflective technique' to generate theory from practice on regular faculty practice days. The issue of faculty practice is another one that has perplexed the profession for quite a time. It is problematic that so much nursing is taught by people who no longer practise, for they are deprived of an important source of nursing knowledge. Their critical reflections on nursing practice are sometimes of a second-hand nature making it difficult for lecturers to gain credibility. Yet the practical problems of faculty practice are complex and mere presence in the workplace is certainly not enough to advance lecturers' knowledge of nursing. Gray & Forsstrom's work (1991) is a useful introduction to reflective practice for lecturers and has great potential for making faculty practice meaningful, besides enabling lecturers to understand the nature of reflective nursing practice which they are encouraging in nursing students. The pertinence of this work will be apparent as lecturers start to nurse therapeutically and are able to reflect critically on their own expertise. They will became therapists when they devise more flexible times and creative methods of practice, offering clients expertise and continuity of service. The nursing academics Snowball, Ross and Murphy (1994) undertook a similarly introspective study to critique and learn about their practice as supervisors of student research.

On a political tack nurses are reviewing their predicament which can appear 'irrational, unjust and unfulfilling' (Emden 1991, p. 348). One example is the exploration of the effects medical dominance has, and has had on the development of the mainly female profession of nursing (Salvage 1985, Lumby 1991, Short, Sharman & Speedy 1992). A critical social view of nursing reveals – through reflection – distortions and inequalities in the system, exposes power relationships and clarifies routes for collaborative change. Nurses are quite aware that in the current political climate they need to understand the complex local, national and international situations of nurses in order to secure a proper contribution in the changing health care system. It is understood that this process of emancipation may well demonstrate the contributions nurses make to their own oppression in the system. However, over a decade after the widespread introduction of critical reflection in undergraduate and postgraduate courses there is little evidence that the broad body of nurses are becoming more politically aware or forceful.

While these reasons for adopting reflection on experience for nursing study are persuasive, some cautions are wisely raised in both nursing and educational literature. These cautions are of a practical, political, philosophical, and moral nature.

It can appear that reflection is easy and something which the students can be sent off to do. However reflection is a process of gradual self-awareness, critical appraisal of the social world and transformation. These are not particularly comfortable processes, which may lead students to personal distress and conflict. Reflective practitioners need handy encouragement and professional help. Most students work with mentors or preceptors, who should understand the process of reflective learning and have been educationally prepared for the role of helping nursing undergraduates. (See the chapters on mentoring, Chapter 4, and clinical supervision, Chapter 5.) Students who only share reflections with faculty members will miss important input from practising nurses who bring a practical balance to the sometimes openly ideological views supported by the academy. The students and mentors should be guided and supported by lecturers, who have an appreciation of the clinical area in question. This is quite a laborious system and it is one that is susceptible to cuts when economies have to be made; a point amply made and discussed in the chapter on assessment and evaluation of reflection, Chapter 3.

There is perhaps a modern tendency to romanticise nursing practice. It is comfortable to imagine that all nurses are the ingenious carers as described by Benner (1984), however it should be remembered that she investigated 'expert practice'. There would be doubtful benefits if reflection on action gave some nurses the excuse to validate their current practice and ignore theory or continuing education altogether. There are nurses who have cruised through their careers picking up knowledge in an effortless and haphazard way and they may incorrectly relate this process to reflection. While some of the knowledge they gain will be practical, their lack of self critique means that in their work they probably propound some myths, unchallenged attitudes and outdated practices too. The process of reflection is hard work and involves a commitment of both time and intellectual effort in order for the practitioner to progress. It is not something done unintentionally or effortlessly.

Griffiths & Tann (1992) raise the issue of political pressure on professions. The notion of learning on the job for teacher education has appealed to politicians and given some of them an excuse to criticise the colleges of education. Ideas are emerging that all students need is a mentor in practice to show them the ropes, therefore the faculty and investment in the colleges can be reduced. Politicians have berated educationalists for being too theoretical and the source of outlandish and unsuccessful experiments in education. Similarly, pressure has been put on nurses to return to basics and turn from academia to the bed side. We regularly hear moves to reintroduce enrolled nurse training and to change skill mix in clinical areas. Moves to increase experiential learning methods to disproportionate levels within the theoretical courses are probably unjustified as the results of learning from experience as reflective practitioners in education and nursing are mainly disappointing to date (Griffiths & Tann 1992, Burnard 1995, Newell 1994). Besides learning through reflection on experience is not purely experiential as Griffiths & Tann (1992) point out – students are still required to study relevant theories and search the literature in order to augment their own thoughts.

Hargreaves (1997) legitimately addresses the issue of informed consent when nursing students use reflection to document some issues that may not be usually recorded in the written form. Disclosure of such information may well be sanctioned within the oral culture of the clinical milieu, yet in educational settings such information about patients' experiences should be viewed as privileged and afforded discretion and respect. Thompson *et al.* (cited by Hargreaves (Hargreaves 1997, p. 225) suggests that 'clinical training without patients... is like learning to swim on dry land'. Nevertheless, the use of patient data, documentation of their feelings and their impact on others, as is the case in reflective 'journalling', is not generally a part of the usual documentation that patients can lawfully view under the freedom of information legislation. Hargreaves (Hargreaves 1997) suggests that a 'priviledged relationship' between the nurse and the patient does not necessarily authorise discussions between the nurse and third parties outside the clinical environment. She admits that this issue has not been addressed in much of the literature on reflection. Rather, the ethical dilemmas posed by such anomalies are largely ignored or contained under the rubric of research etiquette. However, as Hargreaves (1997) argues in research situations patients sign their consent to participate, yet as part of the reflective process they are largely ignorant of the central role they play. That students and lecturers alike should pay heed to the ethical considerations of the reflective process is one way that Hargreaves (1997, p. 227) believes these issues can be addressed. She further attests to the development of a suitably devised 'code of ethics' for reflective practice in nurse education. The use of such a code would, according to Hargreaves be more in keeping with the tenor of emancipation, put forward as a core realisation of critical reflection.

It is apparent that students and quite often lecturers are aware that critical reflection will almost inevitably lead the student to challenge and change the status quo. Even in the early days Oxford nursing students were creating dissonance in both the practice and educational institutions. Some would applaud this as it is about time nurses questioned practice and brought about changes in some traditional spheres. However, it is appropriate to question how fair it is that neophytes are set up to do this difficult work without adequate preparation or indeed authority. Freire (1972) warns of the disillusion experienced by the oppressed, who identify the sources of their oppression and yet are still powerless to make a difference.

Emancipation through critical reflection needs a considerable degree of maturity, for the student is required to reframe personal perspectives – to see situations in new ways, not necessarily always from their perspective. Other parties' points of view need to be considered as fairly as possible in order to build up a comprehensive social picture. It is likely that nurses contribute to their own oppression and the oppression of others. Change in personal perspective (perspective transformation) is required to deal with others in a fair and equitable manner. Premature mounting of personal or professional soap boxes is not a reasonable goal for the critically reflective practitioner, but one we fear may be all too easy to achieve, if care is not taken to avoid this narrow perspective.

So reflection on experience and critical reflection may enable nurses to focus on practice and give it premier status within the discipline. They may find it a useful pathway to the generation and articulation of knowledge, specific and practically useful to nursing in both clinical and academic institutions. It may also provide the means for nurses to understand and contribute towards change in their social world. These are optimistic assertions that should be tempered with caution. Reflection is not a panacea for nursing's many dilemmas – it is a way of learning more about our work. Whatever method is chosen for learning the important factors will always be the individual's ability and commitment to learn and the conduciveness of the learning institution.

Research

It is understandable that there has not been a large evaluative study of the effectiveness of critical reflection as a learning technique in nursing, because in the present political era research funding in health care is usually secured by researchers whose work is directly related to health outcomes. The result of this is that research in the area is made up of disparate, usually small, studies that do not add up to a substantial body of evidence to guide the profession. While it is reasonable to suggest that we cannot have conclusive evidence on which to base all our work, it is questionable to continue a practice that we are not prepared to justify through evaluating its effectiveness and appropriateness.

Nursing has reached a stage where there is an abundance of literature on the subject of critical reflection, however the literature is largely theoretical, speculative or frankly anecdotal and beginning to be repetitive. If they wish to add anything substantive to the topic it is time for new commentators to inject some empirical research into the discourses. As was commented on in an earlier edition of this chapter it is a difficult area to research, bearing in mind the underlying philosophies of critical reflection and the range of ways that critical reflection appears to be used in nursing education. A team of researchers in a major study could approach the subject from a number of angles and throw light on different aspects of reflection, collecting and analysing both qualitative and quantitative data. What research there is tends to be small scale looking at student or teaching staff's perspectives (Burnard 1995, Durgahee 1996), identifying teaching/facilitative processes (Wallace 1996, Durgahee 1998) or assessing students' levels of reflexivity (Richardson & Maltby 1995, Wong, Kember, Chung & Yan 1995). Research studies that show positive results either in students' ability to nurse or patient outcomes as a result of reflective practice as a learning tool are difficult to find.

Durgahee's work does provide information regarding the progress that nursing students from community, psychiatric and hospital settings saw in themselves one year after using reflection as a learning technique on a course (Durgahee 1996, p. 160). In this research 110 nurses were surveyed (80% response rate) and 50 were interviewed to elicit whether the students valued the reflective processes and what the impact of reflective practice was for their practice. The researchers conclude that 'the educational experience has enhanced powers of clinical reasoning.... Through narrative framing of critical incidents, questioning and interacting, students have accumulated cues and patterns which facilitate cognitive reasoning'. The question that is not answered is how this impacts on patient care. As an extension of the original research, Durgahee (1998) investigated the facilitative processes most conducive to learning from reflection. In this study, using the illuminative evaluation model of Parlett & Hamilton (1972), data were collected from participant observation of 60 reflective diary sessions and group interviews with 110 nurses who were undertaking a post-graduate course in care of the dying. In this study resistance to student directed learning was uncovered as were concepts that led to the development of a model for facilitation, namely: purposefulness, activity, collaboration, critical thinking and confrontation and support, PACTS. Investigation into the process of reflection is of course important and work by Johns (1996) and Durgahee (1998) are helpful as they help to establish models that can be used by facilitators and students as guides to help their reflections.

To further explore the research issues, what may be confusing to some is that critical reflection is an integral part of emancipatory or critical enquiry methodologies. Smith (1990, p. 177) lists these methodologies within the critical paradigm as 'critical praxis, research-as-praxis, emancipatory research, action research, and critical ethnography'. These approaches all have components where critical theorems arise from the research participants' critical reflection of the information collected. This process reveals power relationships, particular interests and distortions that compound the particular practical situation under scrutiny. It is argued, albeit in a less deliberate way, that nurses who use critical reflection on their actions, as a method of understanding their work, are akin to researchers generating theories.

Usher (1985), Cox et al. (1991) Griffiths & Tann (1992) and Rolfe (1998) discuss the relationship between personal knowledge generated from individual experience and theories that are derived from literature. Usher (1985, p. 103) explains that they simply represent different perspectives and together knowledge derived in these different ways complements the total view of the problem under scrutiny. Cox et al. (1991, p. 388) agree but proceed further in explaining how theories generated professionally from experience and enacted in the nursing situation are an important contribution to the disciplinary knowledge of nursing. Important because they represent the essential nature of nursing practice. We need more researchers who can interpret these stories and generate theories for use.

Conclusion

Boud & Walker (1991) believe that people need to be able to learn from their experience in order to accept positions of responsibility. The process of learning to learn from experience is as important as the end product of the learning, namely an ability to view a phenomenon from a different perspective and translate new knowledge into action. The process is important because it equips the professional to meet various practical problems and deal with them intelligently – a necessary requirement for all nurses. This is especially so as nursing changes to meet the demands of society into the next millenium. No longer are nurses training to work just in hospitals – they work in many different areas and it is to be hoped that their critical ability will enable them to appraise new work and identify what needs to be learnt, challenged, altered and further investigated in any nursing context.

Reflection on experience is a path that is worth pursuing for it leads in the right direction: towards an education where nurses learn to understand the meaning of their experiences, towards a profession that values its practical expertise, towards a research tradition that has a language that adequately expresses nursing work and finally towards a discipline whose knowledge is not only embedded in nursing practice but can be expressed in new and transforming ways. Part of the pursuit should however be continued research in the area and particularly some evaluation of its effectiveness in achieving, or at least working towards, these ideals and its appropriateness and acceptability to students and facilitators.

References and further reading

Adler, S. (1991) The reflective practitioner and the curriculum of teacher education. *Journal of Education for Teaching*, **17** (2), 139–50.

Alexander, M.F. (1983) *Learning to Nurse*, Churchill Livingstone, Edinburgh.

Argyris, C. & Schön, D. (1974) *Theory in Practice: Increasing Professional Effectiveness*, Jossey-Bass, San Francisco.

Argyris, C. & Schön, D. (1978) *Organisational Learning*, Addison-Wesley, Massachusetts.

Atkins, S. & Murphy, C. (1993) Reflection: a review of the literature. *Journal of Advanced Nursing*, **18** (8), 1188–92.

Bell, L. & Schniedewind, N. (1987) Reflective minds/intentional hearts: joining humanistic education and critical theory for liberating education. *Journal of Education*, **169** (2), 55–78.

Benner, P. (1984) *From Novice to Expert: Excellence and Power in Clinical Nursing Practice*, Addison-Wesley, California.

Benner, P. & Wrubel, J. (1989) *The Primacy of Caring: Stress and Coping in Health and Illness*, Addison-Wesley, California.

Bevis, E. & Watson, J. (1989) *Toward a Caring Curriculum: A New Pedagogy for Nursing*, National League for Nursing, New York.

Boud, D., Keogh, R. & Walker, D. (1985) *Reflection: Turning Experience into Learning*, Kogan Page, London.

Boud, D. & Walker, D. (1991) *Experiencing and Learning: Reflection at Work*, Deakin University Press, Geelong.

Burnard, P, (1995) Nurse educators' perceptions of reflection and reflective practice: a report of a descriptive study. *Journal of Advanced Nursing*, **21**, 1167–74.

Campbell, I. (1992) Myriad – The use of arts as a reflective process in nurse education. Paper presented at the Royal College of Australia First National Nursing Forum, *Nursing Kaleidoscope: Sharpen the Focus*, Adelaide.

Carr, W. & Kemmis, S. (1986) *Becoming Critical: Education, Knowledge and Action Research*, The Falmer Press, London.

Champion, R. (1992) The philosophy of an honours degree program in nursing and midwifery. In Bines, H. & Watson, D. (eds) *Developing Professional Education,*. Society for Research into Higher Education & Open University Press, Milton Keynes.

Clarke, M. (1986) Action and reflection: practice and theory in nursing. *Journal of Advanced Nursing*, **11**, 3–11.

Clarke, B., James, C. & Kelly, J. (1996) Reflective practice: reviewing the issues and refocusing the debate. *International Journal of Nursing Studies*, **33** (20), 181–9.

Clinton, M. (1998) On reflection in action: unaddressed issues in refocusing the debate on reflective practice, *International Journal of Nursing Practice*, **4** (3), 197–203.

Cox, H. & Moss, C. (1988) Promiscuous knowledge: the chaos of practice. The Olive Anstey Nursing Foundation International Conference: *Promiscuous Knowledge*. Perth.

Cox, H., Hickson, P. & Taylor, B. (1991) Exploring reflection: knowing and constructing practice. In Grey, G. & Pratt, R. *Towards a Discipline of Nursing*, Churchill Livingstone, Melbourne.

Deakin University (1988) *Diploma of Nursing: Curriculum. Document*, Deakin School of Nursing, Geelong.

Descartes, R. (1984) The search for truth. In *The Philosophical Writings of Descartes*, Vol. 2, Cottingham, J., Stoothoff, R. & Murdoch, D. (eds) Cambridge University Press, Cambridge.

Dewey, J. (1933) *How We Think*, D.C. Heath, Boston.

Durgahee, T. (1996) Promoting reflection in post-graduate nursing: a theoretical model. *Nurse Education Today*, **16**, 419–26.

Durgahee, T. (1998) Facilitating reflection: from a sage on stage to a guide on the side, *Nurse Education Today*, **18**, 158–64.

Emden, C. (1991) Becoming a reflective practitioner. In Gray, G. & Pratt, R. *Towards a Discipline of Nursing*, Churchill Livingstone, Melbourne.

FitzGerald, M. (1996) The practical implications of a critique of traditional science, *International Journal of Nursing Practice*, **1** (1), 2–12.

Freire, P. (1972) *Pedagogy of the Oppressed*, Penguin Books, Harmondsworth.

Garrison, D. (1991) Critical thinking and adult education: a conceptual model for developing critical thinking in adult learners. *International Journal of Lifelong Education*, **10** (4), 287–303.

George, P. (1986) The nurse as a reflective practitioner. Unpublished paper, Oxford Polytechnic, Oxford.

Giovanetti, P. (1986) Evaluation of Primary Nursing. In Weilty, H., Fitzpatrick, J. & Taundon, J. *The Annual Review of Nursing Research*, Springer Publishing Company, New York.

Glen, S. (1995) Developing critical thinking in higher education, *Nurse Education Today*, **15**, 170–76.

Graham, I.W. (1995), Reflective practice: using the action learning group mechanism, *Nurse Education Today*, **15**, 28–32.

Gray, J. & Forsstrom, S. (1991) Generating theory from practice: the reflective technique. In Gray, G. & Pratt, R. *Towards a Discipline of Nursing*, Churchill Livingstone, Melbourne.

Greenwood, J. (1993) Reflective practice: a critique of the work of Argyris and Schön. *Journal of Advanced Nursing* **18**, 1183–7.

Griffiths, M. & Tann, S. (1992) Using reflective practice to link personal and public theories. *Journal of Education for Teaching*, **18** (1), 69–84.

Habermas, J. (1977) *Knowledge and Human Interests*, Beacon Press, Boston.

Hargreaves, J. (1997) Using patients: exploring the ethical dimensions of reflective practice in nurse education, *Journal of Advanced Nursing*, **25**, 223–8.

Hickson, P. (1988) *Knowledge and action in nursing: a critical approach to the practice worlds of our nurses*. Unpublished Master's Thesis, Massey University, Toronto.

Holly, M. (1987) *Keeping a personal-professional journal*, revised edn, Deakin University Press, Geelong.

Holmes, C. (1991) Theory: where are we going and what have we missed along the way? In Gray, G. and Pratt, R. *Towards a Discipline of Nursing*, Churchill Livingstone, Melbourne.

Johns, C. (1993) On becoming effective in taking ethical action, *Journal of Clinical Nursing*, **2**, 307–12.

Johns, C. (1994a) Guided reflection. In Palmer, A., Burns, S. and Bulman C. (Eds) *Reflective Practice in Nursing: the Growth of the Professional Practitioner*, Blackwell Science, Oxford.

Johns, C. (1994b) *The Burford NDV Model: Caring Practice*, Blackwell Science, Oxford.

Johns, C. (1995) Framing learning through reflection within Carper's fundamental ways of knowing. *Journal of Advanced Nursing*, **22**, 226–34.

Johns, C. (1996) Visualising and realising caring in practice through guided reflection. *Journal of Advanced Nursing*, **24**, 1135–43.

Johns, C. & Freshwater, D. (1998) *Transforming Nursing through Reflective Practice*, Blackwell Science, Oxford.

Kuhn, T. (1970) *The Structure of Scientific Revolutions*, 2nd edn, University of Chicago Press, Chicago.

Laudan, L. (1977) *Progress and Its Problems: Towards a Theory of Scientific Growth*, University of California, Berkeley.

Lawler, J. (1991) *Behind the Screens Nursing Somology, the Problem of the Body*, Churchill Livingstone, Melbourne.

Lumby, J. (1991) Threads of an emerging discipline. In Gray, G. & Pratt, R. *Towards a Discipline of Nursing*, Churchill Livingstone, Melbourne.

Lumby, J. (1992) Re-emergence of vision. Paper presented at The Royal College of Nursing Australia First National Nursing Forum, *Nursing Kaleidoscope: Sharpen the Focus*, Adelaide, June.

Macquarie Dictionary (1991) *The Macquarie Dictionary*, 2nd edn, Macquarie Library Pty Ltd, Sydney.

Menke, E. (1983) Critical analysis of theory development in nursing. In Chaska, N. (ed.) *The Nursing Profession*, McGraw-Hill, New York.

Mezirow, J. (1981) A critical theory of adult learning and education, *Adult Education*, **32** (1), 3–24.

Miller, A. (1985) The relationship between nursing theory and nursing practice. *Journal of Advanced Nursing*, **10**, 414-24.

Munhall, P.L. (1982) Nursing philosophy and nursing research: in apposition or opposition? *Nursing Research*, **31** (3), 176–7, 181.

Murphy, C. & Reading, P. (1992) Assessing professional competence. In Bines, H. & Watson, D. (eds) *Developing Professional Education*, Society for Research into Higher Education & Open University Press, Buckingham.

Newell, R. (1992) Anxiety, accuracy and reflection: the limits of professional development. *Journal of Advanced Nursing*, **17**, 1326–33.

Newell, R. (1994) Reflection: art, science or pseudo-science. Guest Editorial, *Nurse Education Today*, **14**, 79–81.

Oxford Brookes University (formerly Oxford Polytechnic), Department of Nursing, Midwifery and Health Visiting (1988) Submission of course proposals. Unpublished.

Parlett, M. & Hamilton, D. (1972) *Evaluation as Illumination: A New Approach to the Study of Innovatory Programs*. Occasional paper, Centre for Educational Research in Educational Sciences, University of Edinburgh.

Pearson, A. (1988) *Primary Nursing – Nursing in the Burford and Oxford Nursing Development Units*, Croom Helm, London.

Pearson, A. (1991). Nursing as caring. In McMahon, R. & Pearson, A. *Nursing as Therapy*, Chapman & Hall, London.

Pearson, A. (1992) Knowing nursing: emerging paradigms in nursing. In Robinson, K. & Vaughan, B. (eds) *Knowledge for Nursing Practice*. John Wiley, London.

Pearson, A., Whitehouse, C. & Morris, P. (1985) Consumer orientated groups: a new approach to interdisciplinary teaching. *Journal of the Royal College of Practitioners*, **35**, 381–3.

Perry, J. (1985) *Theory & practice in the induction of graduate nurses: a reflexive critique*, Master's Thesis, Massey University, Toronto.

Perry, J. & Moss, C. (1989) Generating alternatives in nursing: turning curriculum into a living process. *The Australian Journal of Advanced Nursing*, **6** (2), 3540.

Powell, J. (1991) Reflection and the evaluation of experience: prerequisites for therapeutic practice. In McMahon, R. & Pearson, A. *Nursing as Therapy*, Chapman & Hall, London.

Richardson, R. (1995) Humpty Dumpty: reflection and reflective nursing practice, *Journal of Advanced Nursing*, **21**, 1044–50.

Richardson, G. & Maltby, H. (1995) Reflection-on-practice: enhancing student learning, *Journal of Advanced Nursing*, **22**, 235–42.

Robinson, K. & Vaughan, B. (1992) *Knowledge for Nursing Practice*, John Wiley, London.

Rolfe, G. (1998) Beyond expertise: reflective and reflexive nursing practice. In Johns C. & Freshwater D. (eds) *Transforming Nursing Through Reflective Practice*. Blackwell Science, Oxford.

Salvage, J. (1985) *The Politics of Nursing*. Heinemann, London.

Sater, B. (1988) *The Stream of Becoming: A Study of Martha Roger's Theory*. National League for Nursing, New York.

Schank, M.J. (1990) Wanted: nurses with critical thinking skills, *The Journal of Continuing Education in Nursing*, **21** (2), 86–9.

Schön, D. (1983) *The Reflective Practitioner*, Basic Books Harper Collins, San Francisco.

Schön, D. (1987) *Educating the Reflective Practitioner*. Jossey-Bass, San Francisco.

Schumacher, K & Gortner, S. (1992) (Mis) conceptions and reconceptions about traditional science. *Advances in Nursing Science*, **14** (4), 1–11.

Shapiro, S. (1991) The end of radical hope? Postmodernism and the challenge to critical pedagogy. *Education and Society*, **9** (2), 112–22.

Shor, I. (1987) *Critical Teaching and Everyday Life*, University of Chicago Press, Chicago.

Short, S., Sharman, E. & Speedy, S. (1992) *Sociology for Nurses*, Macmillan, London.

Silva, M. (1977) Philosophy, science, theory: interrelationships and implications for nursing research. *Image*, **9**, 59–63.

Smith, B. (1990) The critical approach. In Smith, B., Connole, H., Speedy, S. and Wisean, R. *Issues and Methods in Research Study Guide*, South Australian College of Advanced Education, Adelaide.

Smith, P. (1992) *The Emotional Labour of Nursing: How Nurses Care*, Macmillan, London.

Smyth, W. (1986) *Reflection in Action*, Deakin University Press, Geelong.

Snowball, J. Ross, K. & Murphy, C. (1994), Illuminating dissertation supervision through reflection, *Journal of Advanced Nursing*, **19** (6), 1234–40.

Street, A. (1988) *Nursing Practice: High, hard ground, messy swamps and the pathways in between*, Deakin University Press, Geelong.

Street, A. (1992) *Inside Nursing: a Critical Ethnography of Clinical Nursing Practice*, Suny Cornhill.

Turner, B. (1990) *Theories of Modernity and Post Modernity*, Sage Publications, San Mateo.

UKCC (1986) *Project 2000: A New Preparation for Practice*, United Kingdom Central Council for Nursing, Midwifery and Health Visiting, London.

Usher, R. (1985) Beyond the anecdotal: adult learning and the use of experience. *Studies in the Education of Adults*, **17** (1), 59–74.

Wallace, D. (1996) Experiential learning and critical thinking in nursing. *Nursing Standard* **10** (31), 43–7.

Watson, J. (1985) *Nursing – the Philosophy and Science of Caring*, Colorado Associated University Press, Denver.

Wellard, S. J. & Bethune, E. (1996) Reflective journal writing in nurse education: whose interest does it serve? *Journal of Advanced Nursing*, **24**, 1077–82.

Wheeler, C. & Chinn, P. (1991) *Peace and Power: A Handbook of Feminist Process*, 3rd edn, National League for Nurses, New York.

Wong, K., Kember, D., Chung, L. and Yan, L. (1995) Assessing the levels of student reflection from reflective journals *Journal of Advanced Nursing*, **22**, 48–57.

Chapter 2
Developing Underlying Skills in the Move Towards Reflective Practice

Introduction

Certain skills are needed to become a reflective practitioner, in much the same way as it takes good clinical skills to be a competent nurse. The purpose of this chapter is to:

- define and explore some of the skills underlying the use of reflective practice
- enable practitioners to examine, further develop and refine these skills.

Previous work has identified the skills of self awareness, description, critical analysis, synthesis and evaluation as crucial to the use of reflection as an approach to learning from and during professional practice (Atkins & Murphy 1993). Self awareness underpins all good nursing practice, and is essential for establishing effective and therapeutic nurse–patient relationships. Knowing how to describe, analyse, synthesise and evaluate are also important skills for all professional nurses (Schank 1990). While reflection is a natural human thinking process, the deliberate and systematic use of reflection as a learning tool in professional practice is a complex activity. It needs to be consciously developed by students and practitioners over time, and fostered by educators (Boud *et al.* 1985, Schön 1987). A variety of approaches have been shown to be effective in promoting and enhancing reflection, for example the use of a structured framework or model (Johns 1996, Gibbs 1988), and journal writing (Paterson 1995, Richardson & Maltby 1995). The skills based approach presented in this chapter is complementary to these more widely accepted approaches.

This chapter presents a series of exercises, designed for both students and qualified nurses who wish to examine, develop and refine their skills for reflective practice. It is also intended to be of some practical help to educators, clinical supervisors and mentors involved in encouraging and facilitating reflection in others. A separate section is devoted to each skill. The meaning of the skill is defined and explored, with examples of its use in everyday life and professional nursing practice, as well as in academic work. The importance of each skill for reflective practice is justified with reference to key theories. It is also the intention to demystify some of the language and terminology associated with the skills and processes of reflection. The series of exercises will enable participants to practise the skills of reflection alone, with a colleague or friend, and within a group.

The importance of underlying skills

When examining the processes of reflective practice and learning, as identified by key and influential authors, for example Boud *et al.* (1985), Schön (1991) and Mezirow (1981), the importance of underlying skills becomes apparent. Regardless of which theory, model or framework one uses as a guide to reflection, the need for underlying skills is evident to varying degrees. For example, in Boud *et al.*'s (1985) analysis of the reflective process, the need to attend to feelings and attitudes (in particular making use of positive feelings and dealing with negative feelings) is apparent throughout, and requires self awareness. The stages labelled as 'Association', 'Integration', 'Validation' and 'Appropriation' involve varying degrees of critical analysis, synthesis and evaluation. Similarly, if one takes Mezirow's (1981) concept of reflectivity and examines its seven different dimensions or levels, it is clear that self awareness is integral at all levels. The need for description, analysis, synthesis and evaluation becomes more evident as one moves up the hierarchy from 'Discriminant' to 'Theoretical' reflectivity.

It is also interesting to note that the skills required to engage in reflective practice are similar to those required for academic work. With the exception of self awareness, these underlying skills are the higher order cognitive or thinking skills identified within Bloom *et al.*'s (1956) taxonomy of educational objectives. This taxonomy or hierarchy has guided and influenced the development of higher education programmes, learning objectives and outcomes in many different disciplines. It might, therefore, be suggested that the abilities of a reflective practitioner of nursing are not so different from the abilities required by a person engaged in academic pursuits, including research. Developing and refining the underlying skills should, therefore, not only help nurses to become more reflective practitioners, but assist with developing the skills necessary for undertaking further study or courses, and help students integrate reflective writing within academic work.

Reflective practice versus critical thinking

In explaining and discussing some of the language and terminology associated with reflective practice, it may be helpful to examine the relationship between reflective practice and critical thinking. Recently, and with the movement of nursing education into higher education, there has been a growing interest in applying the concept of critical thinking to nursing and nursing education (Brookfield 1993, Daly 1998, Wallace 1996). It is also the case that terms such as critical reflection, critical thinking, critical awareness and critical analysis are sometimes used interchangeably, which may result in a lack of clarity about their meaning and cause confusion.

While some authors emphasise critical thinking as a rational, linear, problem solving process grounded in the scientific approach (Siegal 1988, Fisher 1995), the more widely accepted view appears to be that critical thinking involves an affective dimension; in that acknowledging and analysing feelings is a fundamental and important part of the process (Dewey 1933, Brookfield 1987). This is supported by the ethnographic studies of Brookfield (1993) and Wallace (1996), that explored nurses' critical thinking processes in practice. The findings of both studies suggest that acknowledgement and analysis of feelings and attitudes, that is an emotional component, is important if the outcome of critical thinking is to have a positive effect on learning, nursing development and patient care. Brookfield's (1987) key components of critical thinking: identifying and challenging assumptions and imagining and exploring alternative ways of thinking and acting, are key activities undertaken during the critical analysis phase of a reflective cycle or process. Furthermore, as with reflective practice, it is evident that the notion of critical thinking has been informed by critical social theory (Mezirow 1981). Brookfield (1987) contends that critical thinking is necessary for healthy relationships, effective work and political activity. It would seem, therefore, that although the processes of reflective practice and critical thinking are similar, the term reflective practice does convey an approach to professional practice which is not only concerned with thinking, but also with the acknowledgement of feelings and with activity that makes a positive difference to practice. In conclusion, it may be helpful to refer to Reid's definition of reflective practice: 'a process of reviewing an experience of practice in order to describe, analyse and evaluate and so inform learning from practice' (Reid 1993, p. 305).

Guidance on using the exercises in this chapter

When undertaking the following exercises, their limitations need to be understood. First, reflective practice skills are acquired and developed gradually through practice over time, rather than in any one course or package (see Sue Duke's chapter, Chapter 7, on becoming reflective). While these exercises involve reflecting on practice, frequently away from the clinical setting, it should be acknowledged that reflective practice, most importantly, is a way of reviewing practice while engaged in the actual delivery of nursing care. Second, people learn in different ways, and the extent to which individuals find this skills based approach to developing reflective practice useful will depend upon their general approach to learning. Third, it needs to be recognised that there may be other skills, not addressed in this chapter, which can help people to develop reflective practice.

Three types of exercises are presented. They are:

- On-your-own exercises. It is recommended to take about 15–30 minutes with these exercises.
- With-a-partner exercises. These exercises usually take approximately 30–60 minutes.
- With-a-group exercises. These exercises usually take between 30–90 minutes.

All exercises require a commitment of time and thought. Taking the exercises slowly over several weeks is recommended as the best approach. When developing your skills it may also be helpful to refer to the many examples and extracts of reflection within other chapters of this book.

Issues for facilitators

It is recommended that facilitators be educators or clinical supervisors with experience of working with adult learners. Ground rules will need to be established when working with a group. Facilitators need to be reflective practitioners themselves. Scanlan and Chernomas (1997) suggest that many nurse educators have undertaken educational programmes in which reflective strategies were not identified explicitly. It may be the case, therefore, that their understanding of reflection is based on experiences with students and reading of the literature rather than their own conscious experiences with reflection. Facilitators can prepare themselves by following the guidelines below.

- Review all exercises from a personal point of view, as well as from an educational perspective. If you have not had the opportunity to engage in the exercises as a participant prior to being a facilitator, it is important that you at least challenge yourself with the on-your-own exercises.

- Be prepared to role model or participate in all exercises. It is essential that the facilitator demonstrates an openness and willingness to share experiences. Reflecting on experiences may be seen as risky by participants. Facilitators can best provide support and encouragement by example.

- Co-facilitation is highly recommended, where possible and depending on the size of the group. With more than one facilitator, participants can benefit by the increased accessibility of a facilitator. The facilitators can also benefit by the opportunity for ongoing dialogue and reflection with a peer.

- Bearing in mind the limitations of such a programme of exercises, and the fact that they are in no way intended to be comprehensive, facilitators should be prepared to guide participants to further appropriate resources.

Self awareness

To be self aware is to be conscious of one's character, including beliefs, values, qualities, strengths and limitations. It is about knowing oneself. Burnard (1992) distinguishes between the inner self, how one feels inside, and the outer self, the aspects that other people see, including appearance, verbal and non-verbal behaviour.

Self awareness is the foundation skill upon which reflective practice is built. It underpins the entire process of reflection, because it enables people to see themselves in a particular situation and honestly observe how they have affected the situation and how the situation has affected them. Self awareness also enables a person to analyse his or her feelings, which is an essential component of reflection. It is evident from influential research and theoretical work that it is the use of self awareness and self or personal knowledge which differentiates reflective learning from other types of mental activity, for example logical thinking and problem solving (Boud *et al.* 1985, Mezirow 1981).

It is important, although obvious, to state that self awareness is necessary, not only for reflective learning, but for skilled professional nursing practice. Knowledge of one's own beliefs, values and behaviour, and how these affect others is essential for developing good interpersonal skills and building therapeutic relationships with patients. In addition, all adult learners need to be self aware to enable them to take responsibility for identifying and responding to their learning needs, and to develop greater independence in initiating, planning, conducting and communicating work, whether in relation to formal study, or professional lifelong learning.

In some ways, self awareness is hard to avoid, as self interest is part of human nature. However, developing an honest self awareness is more complex. It is natural to want to see and portray ourselves in the most favourable light, and this desire together with our own prejudices and assumptions can sometimes interfere with our ability to take a more objective look at ourselves. Being honest about oneself therefore requires courage, confidence, a certain degree of maturity, and the support of others. In particular, to develop and maintain an appropriate level of self awareness in the work situation and for reflective practice requires substantial effort and mental energy. One is sometimes dealing with deeply held values and strong feelings which may be uncomfortable and anxiety provoking. There will, therefore, be times when one chooses to avoid the process, and when it is becomes more appropriate just to go home and relax. It is, however, important to bear in mind that identifying and releasing one's feelings, both positive and negative, is generally better for a person, provided that the time and place are appropriate. While a degree of personal insight and self awareness is necessary to engage in reflective practice it is also important to recognise that too much negative introspection and analysis can have an adverse effect. There is therefore a need to gain the right balance in any situation.

The following series of exercises aim to help you to identify and clarify beliefs, values and feelings. There are also exercises enabling you to examine your motivation for developing a more reflective type of practice, and the degree to which you are open and receptive to new ideas. These factors have been identified as essential pre-requisites for reflective practice (Dewey 1933, Boud *et al.* 1985).

On-your-own exercise: clarifying values   *15 mins*

A personal value can be described by a statement that says what is important and significant to you as an individual. Describe three of your own values below by completing this sentence:
It is important to me that...

(1)

(2)

(3)

With-a-partner exercise: exploring values   *30 mins*

- Are you clear and certain about what your values are? Give examples. Identify some values that are key for you.
- Do your values always guide your actions? Give examples of when they have done and when they have not.
- How did you acquire the key values in your life? Identify specific people or situations that have affected your values.

Go over the answers to these questions with a partner. Consider how you can become clearer about your own values.

Values perform an important function for everyone. They provide a clear framework for deciding upon a position and they provide a basis for action. Being clear about your values in professional practice will help you to live with the results of your actions. What is interesting about values is that they are chosen but they are not necessarily consistent with one another.

On-your-own exercise: how motivated am I?   *15 mins*

Think about the reasons why you are developing and using reflection. Make a list of these.

You may have identified some good reasons. In addition to enabling you to develop and enhance your nursing practice, reflection is important within formal professional courses, and when profiling learning for professional registration purposes or for the assessment and accreditation of prior experiential learning (APEL). If, however, you believe you have little to gain personally or professionally you may find it more difficult to devote the necessary time. There is always the possibility that this is not the right approach for you or that this is not the right time for you to undertake the exercises.

On-your-own exercise: am I open to new ideas?   *30 mins*

Identify from your professional practice a situation where a colleague introduced a change that would or did have implications for your own practice.

- Describe what the change was.
- What were the significant background factors to this change?
- What were your thoughts about it?
- Identify your feelings about the change.
- How receptive were you to the change? Why was this?
- What were your prejudices and biases?

This exercise may have highlighted two issues. First, change may not be necessarily for the better. It may be that if you had negative feelings towards the change, and that this was because you did not see the change as in the best interests of the team or patients. It may be that you felt that there was insufficient evidence to support the change. Second, you may find change in itself difficult. If so, you need to consider carefully the reasons why. Changes can make people feel insecure and unsettled. There may also be some times in your life when you are more receptive to change than at other times. It is, however, important to remember that openness to new ideas is necessary to be a reflective practitioner.

On-your-own exercise: your life map   *15–30 mins*

On a large piece of paper draw a map or diagram that represents the background and history of your nursing practice or training. Include as much detail as possible. Putting your nursing practice into a picture format may seem awkward or difficult at first, but it will allow you to see your career from a very different perspective. Don't worry about drawing things correctly, just try to be creative.

Include as many of the following events as possible:

- your starting point
- achievements
- joys
- sadnesses
- important people
- obstacles.

With-a-partner exercise: directions and destinations   *30–60 mins*

Take turns explaining the map of your career in nursing or your experiences as a nursing student. Give as much detail as possible, so that your partner can understand your background.

When listening to your partner, pay close attention to the details. Ask questions to better understand your partner's experiences. Also listen for what is left out of your partner's story. Here are some questions you may want to use to probe a little deeper.

- Where are you on your own map? How active or passive are you?
- Where are the strongest emotions on your map? What are these emotions? Have any emotionally strong experiences been left out?
- Are there any other people on your map? Who are they? Is anyone missing who should be there?
- Are there patients on your map? Why or why not?
- What takes up the most space on your map? Why do you think it does?
- Are there any empty spaces on your map? Should something else be included in those spaces? Is there any meaning in the emptiness?

Group exercise: looking for the cross-roads　*30–60 mins*

All participants should post their 'maps' on the walls of the room. Without describing or analysing the maps, look for what is common:

- themes
- symbols
- depictions
- colour choices
- any developments or sequences (e.g. from left to right, bottom to top).

Given the fact that members of the group have lived through similar times and are engaged in the same profession, it isn't surprising that there may be common areas. Value the shared experiences since they can bind the group together and also provide support. Look also for the differences between the 'maps'. These unique versions are valuable to the group in a different way in providing new perspectives. Spend a few minutes talking about the experience of 'mapping'. Allow each participant a chance to answer the question: 'What was the biggest surprise or insight you gained from your own or others' life maps?'

Doing life maps reminds us of the positive aspects of our careers, but it will also bring to mind the low points or sadnesses that we have experienced. Be prepared to support members of the group who need it.

Description

To describe something, whether it be a person, an object, a situation or an abstract concept or idea, is to state its characteristics or appearance without expressing a judgement. A descriptive account is usually in spoken or written form, but may also be in other forms, such as a painting or sculpture.

In appreciating the qualities and power of good description, examples of excellent descriptive accounts are widely available within English literature, both prose and poetry. In particular, the reader is referred to Styles and Moccia's (1993) anthology entitled *On Nursing: a Literary Celebration* which contains many rich descriptive accounts of nursing, and people's experiences of health and illness. Good descriptive abilities are necessary, for example, when communicating with colleagues about patients and for writing clear and accurate patient progress notes. When using reflection, description is the skill with which you recollect the important events and features of your practice. Good description is about giving a clear, accurate and comprehensive account of a situation. The account will include the following key elements: significant background factors (the context), the events as they unfolded in the situation, what you were thinking at the time, how you were feeling at the time, and the outcome of the situation. Your description should reconstruct the situation to enable someone who was not there to understand the situation from your position. What you are trying to do is paint a clear, vivid colourful picture which then allows yourself and possibly others to review the situation.

Some people are gifted with the skill of description while others struggle to find the most appropriate words. A full vocabulary is necessary to be able to describe situations accurately, but at the same time there is a need to avoid the use of jargon and terminology which the reader or listener may not understand and to discriminate between relevant and irrelevant information. A good descriptive account, therefore, demonstrates a full and clear understanding of the relevant and important issues, is well structured and is concise.

Within a piece of written reflection, or when engaging in reflection with another person or a group, it is also important to achieve a balance between description of the situation and the analytical processes which follow. In particular, when undertaking work for academic purposes, it is the higher order thinking skills of analysis and evaluation which are valued, although it is more difficult to engage in these processes without good underlying descriptive skills.

On-your-own exercise: the power of description   *30 mins*

Choose a page of literature from a favourite text, for example a novel, autobiography or poem. Read it carefully. When you feel that you are really familiar with the passage, write down:

● key elements of the description which capture the essence of the situation
● important words or phrases that facilitated your understanding.

It is important to consider what the elements of good description are. If you are able to incorporate these into your writing, you are more likely to give the comprehensive account that enables you to demonstrate your learning through experience. A good piece of description paints a clear and vivid picture of a unique situation. It enables the reader to understand the situation from the writer's perspective. The description contains details which capture not only the significant background factors, but also bring to life these situations through the use of carefully selected words.

On-your-own exercise: I remember when ...   *30 mins*

Identify a work situation in which you were involved recently. The situation might include one or more of the following features:

● you felt that your actions made a real difference to a patient or group of patients
● it went unusually well
● it did not go as planned
● it was very ordinary and typical of your nursing practice
● it captures the essence of what your nursing practice is about.

Take some time to think about the situation. Bearing in mind the features of good description, write down as many of the details that you can remember. There is no need to write in the specific names of people or places involved. Be sure to include information on the following:

● where and when the situation occurred
● who was involved in the situation
● the specific circumstances of the care provided/not provided
● how you felt about the situation at the time
● what you did at the time of the situation
● how you coped after the situation
● what you thought and felt about the situation at a later time.

With-a-partner exercise: 'Let me tell you about ...'   *30–60 mins*

Using your notes from the on-your-own exercise, tell your partner of your experience. Don't be limited by what you wrote. Use your notes as a starting point. When listening to your partner, pay close attention to the details. Ask questions to better understand your partner's experiences. Also listen for what is left out of your partner's story. You may want to probe a little deeper. In telling this story did you talk more about what you felt, thought, and did, or did you describe the actions and attitudes of others?

To facilitate another person's understanding of a situation, you need to give all the relevant factors in enough detail. A common problem may be that because you were involved in the situation, you may omit certain details that you have taken for granted. You may also find it difficult to recall all the key factors in the situation because you have to rely on your memory. It is likely that the situations you will be most able to describe are those which occurred more recently. Sometimes it is important that you can describe situations from your nursing practice, even through they may have occurred some time ago. Keeping a diary that records and describes events in your professional practice may therefore enhance your descriptive abilities.

On-your-own exercise: describing feelings   *30 mins*

Think of a situation in your professional practice where the outcomes were not what you expected or you felt uncomfortable about them. Describe the situation using the elements of good description, then answer the following questions:

- Does your description capture the essence of the situation?
- Does what you have written describe your feelings accurately and truthfully?

It is not always easy to describe feelings you have. Some people find it easier to describe their thoughts about a situation rather than their feelings. When feelings are strong, for example, when we are very happy or very upset, they tend to be easier to acknowledge. However, in any situation there are likely to be feelings beneath the surface that may need more detailed exploration to uncover. Some people find it easier to express feelings than others. If this is true for you, you need to consider some of the reasons why this might be the case. It is generally believed that we are better off identifying and releasing feelings (Boud *et al.* 1985, Boyd & Fales 1983).

On-your-own exercise: judging your description   *30 mins*

This exercise is designed to enable you to judge how effective your skills of description are. Take the description you wrote in one of the previous exercises. Award yourself up to five points for each statement. The maximum score would be 15.

- My description captures the situation accurately.
- My feelings were accurately and honestly reported.
- The key elements are concisely presented.

Look at your score, what were your particular strengths and weaknesses? Some people find it easier to describe facts rather than feelings. An awareness of the difficulties you have will allow you to focus on these and build skills further. If your score fell below 6, you may need to consider repeating these exercises.

Group exercise: my career – the film   *30–90 mins*

Having had an opportunity to get an overview of your career or background, as well as a close up look at a significant incident, you are now in the position of being able to step back for a 'big screen' picture. Ask each member of the group to consider the statement below:

If I were to make a film version of this episode of my career, it would most appropriately be entitled . . .

Feel free to borrow or improvise from existing films or to make up your own title.

Write the answer on a yellow 'sticky' or index card. Ask each member to paste the film title on to a large piece of paper or poster board in the room. As people put up their titles they should explain the reasons for their choice. People may group their titles with those of a similar nature (adventure films, action, disaster, etc.).

Imagining our careers as films may at first seem silly but it can be enjoyable and worthwhile. It also allows the imaginative parts of our brains to put together the disparate pieces of our life into an image that is easier to understand and describe to others.

Critical analysis

Critical analysis is a key skill for both professional practice and academic work. Analysis involves the separation of a whole into its component parts. To analyse something, whether an object, a set of ideas or a situation, is to undertake a detailed examination of the structure or constituent parts or elements and ask questions about them, in order to more fully understand their nature and how the parts relate to and influence each other. The term 'critical' introduces a further dimension to analysis, in that judgements are made about the strengths and weaknesses of the different parts, as well as of the whole. Being critical does have some negative connotations when it is used in everyday life, in that it is a term often associated with finding fault. However, engaging in critical analysis, or undertaking a critique of something is a positive and constructive process because it is about identifying strengths as well as weaknesses. Examples of critical analysis in nursing practice include assessing the condition of a patient, picking up cues and identifying patient problems.

As a professional nurse, the situations you are involved in are unique, and therefore the knowledge that you need in order to understand and solve problems in practice will depend upon the individual components of the situation, in particular the context. It is also important to recognise that any situation will be influenced by your own feelings, attitude and behaviour. When engaging in reflective practice, therefore, the skill of critical analysis involves the following activities:

- identifying and illuminating existing knowledge of relevance to the situation
- exploring feelings about the situation and the influence of these
- identifying and challenging assumptions made
- imagining and exploring alternative courses of action.

Identifying existing knowledge

The knowledge required to understand the situation needs to be identified and scrutinised. You may find that in order to shed light on a particular situation, you need to search for and examine other knowledge that at first may not have seemed relevant. It is therefore important that you identify the types and sources of knowledge that you use in your professional nursing practice. Nursing knowledge has been classified in a number of different ways, and while recognising that any classification is artificial, and that different types of knowledge are interdependent, it is sometimes helpful to refer to a framework or classification when examining one's own knowledge. Several authors distinguish between 'know-how', which consists of practical skills and expertise, and 'know-that', which is theoretical knowledge and knowledge generated through research (Benner 1984, Meleis 1985). According to Robinson (1991), knowledge may be gained from three main sources: personal experience, known as experiential knowledge, social groups (cultural knowledge), and formally, from theory and research (formal knowledge). The work of Carper (1978) has been influential, and is used by Johns (1995) in his 'Structured Model of Reflection'. Carper (1978) identifies four fundamental patterns of knowing from an analysis of the structure of nursing knowledge:

- empirical knowledge – the factual, descriptive and theoretical knowledge, often developed through research
- aesthetic knowledge – gained more subjectively, through unique and particular situations, and sometimes referred to as the art of nursing
- personal knowledge – knowledge of self, used for example in building therapeutic relationships with patients and in helping them cope with illness
- ethical knowledge – concerned with understandings and judgements of what is right, wrong or ought to be done in different situations.

Engaging in a thorough critical analysis involves actively seeking out the ideas, theories and research of others. It is about raising questions such as what do we know and how do we know it?

Exploring feelings related to the situation

In reflective practice, it is necessary to gain an appropriate balance between the more objective activity of analysing thoughts and knowledge, and the analysis of feelings. It is also important to focus on positive feelings as well as trying to deal with negative feelings, in order for the process to be constructive (Boud *et al.* 1985). What needs to be remembered, however, is that the overall purpose of reflection is to contribute to improvements and further developments in patient care. It is the feelings and experiences of patients that are of central concern. Analysis of one's own feelings should not become a self centred or self indulgent activity, but a process which one engages in only so far as it affects and illuminates practice situations, and enhances learning from those situations.

Identifying and challenging assumptions

Identifying assumptions is about recognising when information is taken for granted or presented as fact without the supporting evidence. It is about not taking things at face value. When analysing a situation it may be helpful to ask questions like 'what is being taken for granted here?' and 'how do I know that I've got an accurate picture of the situation? It is easy to carry on through our working and personal lives with the same set of assumptions, beliefs and values about ourselves, about nursing practice and the profession in general. However, there is a need to challenge these assumptions regularly, and to question where they have come from. Challenging the relevance of the context is particularly important. Everything that happens does so in a certain cultural context, so we need to be able to examine the ideas of people from different cultures within the context of our own. Assuming that ideas and practices which work in one cultural context can automatically be carried to another can cause problems. Examples of such difficulties have sometimes been evident in the application of North American nursing models to British nursing systems.

In identifying and challenging assumptions, we become sceptical of claims to universal truth. We do not take things as read. Simply because a practice has existed for a long time does not mean that it is most appropriate for all time or for the moment. Just because an idea is accepted by everybody else does not mean that we have to believe in its innate truth without first checking its correspondence with reality as we experience it (Brookfield 1987).

Challenging the assumptions underlying our own ideas and those of others can be an uncomfortable and intimidating process. It may involve asking awkward questions. It is therefore important to raise awareness, prompt, nurture and encourage the process without making people feel threatened or patronised.

Imagining and exploring alternative courses of action

Central to this is the idea of constantly looking for new ways of doing things and new ways of thinking. Such new ways of living allow for creativity and growth as opposed to routine and stasis. You could ask yourself the following questions: Do I still work in the same way as I did two years ago? Is that appropriate? What if anything do I want to do about that? This aspect of critical analysis also requires one to look at perspectives other than one's own.

On-your-own exercise: analysing your knowledge   *30 mins*

Take a situation previously described. Think about the knowledge that has enabled you to understand the situation. Write a detailed account of relevant knowledge and indicate the sources of the knowledge.

Some of the knowledge you have used is likely to have been gained through personal experience. Remember that while this is a useful and valid way of gaining knowledge, you need to explore the extent to which this knowledge helps you understand the situation. Some knowledge may have been gained through trial and error. It is particularly important to question this knowledge and its limited value. In professional practice, formal knowledge must be a key source of knowledge, and your account should include research-based knowledge where appropriate. If you have been unable to identify any formal sources of knowledge, it may be that you need to do some further thinking and reading. Group or cultural knowledge can be more difficult to identify, as this knowledge is often implicit in everyday practice. It may be taken for granted or be bound up in the assumptions that underlie your practice. It is important that you explore any assumptions made.

With-a-partner exercise: discussing your knowledge   *30-60 mins*

Ask a partner to read the situation you described previously. Discuss together the knowledge which each of you considers is relevant to understanding the situation.

- Was the knowledge that your partner identified the same or different from yours?
- If different, explore the reasons why.
- Agree with your partner which knowledge was most important for understanding the situation.
- Try to identify together any new knowledge that would be relevant to the situation, and suggest alternative knowledge which may give new insights.

On-your-own exercise: analysing your feelings   *30 mins*

Taking a situation described previously, identify any excerpts that involved feelings. Read through the excerpt carefully. Note whether you have identified your feelings where appropriate. If not, why not? Try to explore honestly why you felt the way you did.

If necessary, try again to identify your feelings. Taking the relevant excerpt, think carefully and identify the feelings which were important in that situation. This may include feelings you had within the situation and about it, the feelings you had at the time and the feelings you have now.

Answer the following questions:

- Why did you feel the way you did?
- What are the relevant elements that made you feel that way?
- Was there anything relevant in your past experiences which led you to feel the way you did?

With-a-partner exercise: talking about feelings   *30 mins*

Talk through your feelings with someone you trust.

Reflective practice does involve an analysis of feelings, and without this understanding you may miss real opportunities in your experience to learn about yourself. Increasing self awareness and ability to analyse your feelings will give you insights that may enhance your nursing practice. While analysis of feelings is difficult, if you have not been able to undertake this exercise, you need to consider carefully the reasons why.

On-your-own exercise: 'One way of looking at it' *30 mins*

Critically analyse a situation previously described, from as many different perspectives as possible. Try to imagine the point of view of patients, colleagues and other people who were involved in the situation.

With-a-partner exercise: 'Different ways of looking at it' *30–60 mins*

Practise taking opposing opinions on the situation presented in the previous exercise. Try defending a perspective that is not your own. Support your views with formal knowledge or theory where possible.

Frequently health care professionals operate from substantially different viewpoints. When a dilemma presents itself, practitioners react differently according to their beliefs and principles. The resulting conflict can be both upsetting and baffling. It may be hard to understand how equally concerned caregivers can have opposing opinions.

Group exercise: the great debate *30–90mins*

Divide the group into several teams, depending on the size of the group. Each team should identify and will then represent a key theory used in professional nursing practice. The teams should be asked to debate the following question:

'What theory provides the most value to health care providers?'

Team members should work together to develop their arguments. One or two members of the team should be selected as spokespersons for the group.
Round 1 – each team is allowed five minutes to state the reason why their theory is the most useful to health care providers.
Round 2 – each team is given five minutes to state the reasons why the other theories presented are inadequate in meeting the needs of health care providers.
Success of the teams will be based on the clarity of their communication and arguments.

Synthesis

Synthesis is defined by the *Oxford Dictionary* as 'the process or result of building up separate elements, especially ideas, into a connected and coherent whole'. It could be described as the opposite of analysis.

Synthesis is about being creative, and sometimes may involve original thinking. In professional nursing practice, a patient care plan is an example of the synthesis of information from a variety of different sources. A good care plan is unique to the particular patient and is also dynamic.

In reflective practice synthesis is the ability to integrate new knowledge, feelings or attitudes with previous knowledge, feelings or attitudes. This is necessary in order to develop a fresh insight or a new perspective on a situation and therefore to learn from it. The skill of synthesis is necessary in order to achieve a satisfactory outcome from reflection. This may include the clarification of an issue, the development of a new attitude or way of thinking about something, the resolution of a problem, a change in behaviour or a decision. Such changes may be small or large. New knowledge may potentially be generated, and original ideas or fresh ways of approaching problems or answering questions may be developed. Synthesis involves making choices with regard to relating new ideas to one's past beliefs and values. This is not necessarily an easy process and may seem like trying to fit a square peg into a round hole, depending upon the scope of adjustment being made. Not choosing to incorporate new ideas is choosing to maintain the old. This is not necessarily right or wrong. Changing old ideas should not be done indiscriminately. The important point is that the choice is an informed decision.

The skill of synthesis can be a difficult one. Listening to the way others have put the pieces together in relation to different situations may be helpful at this point.

On-your-own exercise: 'Dear friend...'   *30 mins*

Take some time to think about what you have learned from the previous exercises and write a letter to a friend, real or imagined, telling of the changes you have experienced. Be sure to include some of the following:

● Give an update on yourself and your self awareness – Has it changed? What did you learn by mapping out your career and talking it over with a partner?
● Describe one of the situations that you believe has most influenced your practice.
● Include information about any knowledge or theory you believe has most relevance to your practice.
● Finish off by writing about what you intend to do differently in identifying and handling some of the issues you encounter in your practice.

With-a-partner exercise: spotlight on you *30–60 mins*

In addition to the written reflections that you have undertaken during these exercises, you now have the opportunity to make a video. By recording your thoughts on video you will be able to hear and see yourself express your views about your nursing practice. You will also be able to use the video recording as a yardstick against which to measure your professional growth in the future. On completion, the videotape will be yours alone. There will be no need to share it with anyone other than your partner for the exercises. However, you may choose to show it to a facilitator, friend, family member or mentor, or you may decide to view it again in the privacy of your own home.

You have done all the preparation for this experience in the previous exercises. There is no need to use notes or check your readings. Your partner will prompt you with the questions listed below:

(1) Tell me a little bit about who you are. (Remember the information that you put in the map of your career. You may wish to add to that information.)

(2) Think of a meaningful incident in your professional career. Tell me:

 ● what your role was
 ● what were the choices that you had
 ● what was the choice you made
 ● how you felt about your choice.

(You do not need to use the incident you describe previously in the section on description. Discussion of that incident may have brought to mind other situations that you have faced in practice.)

(3) Where and what type of work you would like to see yourself doing? What changes and improvements would you make in the way you approach and handle the issues that you face?

Try answering these questions in the following time frames:

 ● one year goals
 ● five year goals
 ● end of practice goals.

The idea of videotaping yourself may be intimidating. You may wonder if it is necessary. One of the reasons you are strongly encouraged to videotape yourself in this session is that it allows you the rare opportunity of seeing yourself. Unlike home videos in which the emphasis is on how you look, this video will focus on what you say and how you say it. You will be able to see yourself as others see you and gain a different perspective on yourself. A video, unlike a written account, is more spontaneous allowing you to say what is on your mind without worrying about punctuation or grammar.

Group exercise: the video experience   *30-90 mins*

Looking at ourselves in pictures or on videotape can be an unnerving experience that many approach with fear and others simply avoid. Having just created a videotape of yourself, it is a good time to discuss the experience. As a group, try to take a look at the benefits and risks of having been videotaped. Each participant should independently write down all the advantages and all the disadvantages that videotaping presents. Then going around the room, each participant should mention one plus and one minus about the video that has not yet been mentioned by the other participants. Keep circling the group until all items on everyone's list have been mentioned.

Listing all the pluses and minuses on a flip chart will give participants a 'master list'. Reviewing this complete list will allow individuals, as well as the group to make a final decision on the merits of videotaping. You may find that this discussion will give you new ideas on how you can review and use your videotape in the future.

Evaluation

Evaluation is the ability to make a judgement about the value of some-thing. It entails a 'looking back'. Judgements are often made with reference to pre-defined criteria or standards, for example when assessing the value of a research report or when determining whether or not a patient has achieved certain goals. Evaluation is a high level skill in both reflective practice and academic work. Unfortunately, the idea of evaluation can make people feel uncomfortable, because of its asso-ciation with examinations, performance appraisals and other assess-ments. The fear of being judged badly may make people want to avoid it altogether.

Self assessment or evaluation is a personal process in which we examine ourselves, frequently over time. This is an important compo-nent of reflective nursing practice and professional education. While we can receive input from others and include their observations and opi-nions, ultimately we must judge ourselves. Nurses can frequently be their own toughest critics. Evaluation should not be self torture for past problems. Rather it is future orientated, for example it may involve finding discrepancies between what we say or what we need and what we do in order to make necessary changes. Autobiographies often contain interesting examples of self evaluation, showing how people look back on their lives.

On-your-own exercise: listening to yourself and others   *15–30 mins*

Play back your own or, with permission, your partner's video. Listen to what you or your partner say on the videotape and take notes on the following:

- beliefs/values
- problems to overcome
- goals for the future.

With-a-partner exercise: learning from the past and looking to the future   *30–60mins*

Review with your partner the notes that you have made about the video. Ask your partner if he or she agrees with each of the items you have put into the categories of beliefs/values, problems to overcome, and goals for the future.

After the discussion with your partner, change any of the items if necessary. Use the rest of the time with your partner identifying the following:

- ongoing support systems
- ongoing strategies
- outlook for the next year's practice.

Group exercise: closure   *30–90 mins*

For the last gathering of the group, it is good to look back on the experience, look forward, and look inward at the group. This session should be a time to review and acknowledge all the hard work that went into the exercises. This last session should be personalised by the group in a way that participants feel most appropriate to their experience.

Conclusion

The intention of this chapter has been to raise awareness of key skills underlying reflective practice, and to encourage and support nurses in assessing and developing these skills. It is evident that these skills are not discrete and separate elements, but are inter-related parts of a whole process. While breaking down the process of reflective practice into constituent parts may be helpful as an educational strategy, the challenge comes with combining and integrating the different elements. This is essential, not only for producing well balanced reflective accounts, but for developing an approach to professional nursing practice, or a way of thinking, whereby one constantly reviews practice in order to learn and to improve standards of care.

References

Atkins, S. & Murphy, K. (1993) Reflection: a review of the literature. *Journal of Advanced Nursing*, **18**, 1188–92.

Benner, P. (1984) *From Novice to Expert: Excellence and Power in Clinical Nursing Practice*, Addison-Wesley, Menlo Park, CA.

Bloom, B.S., Englehart, M.D., Furst, E.J., Hill, W.H. & Krathwohl, D.R. (1956) *Taxonomy of Educational Objectives, Handbook 1: Cognitive Domain*, Longman, London.

Boud, D., Keogh, R. & Walker, D. (1985) Promoting reflection in learning: a model. In Boud, D., Keogh, R. & Walker, D. (eds) *Reflection: Turning Experience into Learning*, Kogan Page, London, pp. 18–39.

Boyd, E.M. & Fales, A.W. (1983) Reflective learning: key to learning from experience. *Journal of Humanistic Psychology*, **23** (2), 99–117.

Brookfield, S.D. (1987) *Developing Critical Thinkers: Challenging Adults to Explore Alternative Ways of Thinking and Acting*, Open University Press, Milton Keynes.

Brookfield, S. (1993) On impostorship, cultural suicide and other dangers: how nurses learn critical thinking. *The Journal of Continuing Education in Nursing*, **23** (5), 197-205.

Burnard, P. (1992) *Know Yourself! Self-awareness Activities for Nurses*, Scutari Press, Harrow.

Carper, B. A. (1978) Fundamental patterns of knowing in nursing. *Advances in Nursing Science–Practice Orientated Theory*, **1** (1), 13–23.

Daly, W.H. (1998) Critical thinking as an outcome of nursing education. What is it? Why is it important to nursing practice? *Journal of Advanced Nursing*, **28** (2), 323–31.

Dewey, J. (1933) *How We Think*, D. C. Heath and Co, Boston.

Fisher, A. (1995) *Infusing Critical Thinking into the College Curriculum*, Centre for Research in Critical Thinking, UEA, Norwich.

Gibbs, G. (1988) *Learning by Doing: A guide to teaching and learning methods*, Further Education Unit, Oxford Polytechnic (*now* Oxford Brookes University), Oxford.

Johns, C.C. (1995) Framing learning through reflection with Carper's fundamental ways of knowing. *Journal of Advanced Nursing*, **22**, 226–34.

Johns, C. C. (1996) Using a reflective model of nursing and guided reflection. *Nursing Standard*, **11** (2), 34–8.

Meleis, A. (1985) *Theoretical Nursing: Development and Progress*, Lippincott, Philadelphia.

Mezirow, J. (1981) A critical theory of adult learning and education. *Adult Education*, **32** (1), 3–24.

Paterson, B.L. (1995) Developing and maintaining reflection in clinical journals. *Nurse Education Today*, **15**, 211–20.

Reid, B. (1993) 'But we're doing it already!' Exploring a response to the concept of reflective practice in order to improve its facilitation. *Nurse Education Today*, **13**, 305–9.

Richardson, G. & Maltby, H. (1995) Reflection-on-practice: enhancing student learning. *Journal of Advanced Nursing,* **22**, 235–42.

Robinson, K. (1991) What we know and how do we know it? (i) Types of knowledge. *Nursing Times,* **87** (20), viii.

Scanlan, J.M. & Chernomas, W.M. (1997) Developing the reflective teacher. *Journal of Advanced Nursing,* **25**, 1138–43.

Schön, D. (1987) *Educating the Reflective Practitioner,* Jossey Bass, San Francisco.

Schön, D. (1991) *The Reflective Practitioner,* 2nd edn, Jossey Bass, San Francisco.

Scriven, M. & Fisher, A. (1994) *Defining and Assessing Critical Thinking,* Sage, London.

Schank, M.J. (1990) Wanted: nurses with critical thinking skills. *The Journal of Continuing Education in Nursing,* **21** (2), 86–9.

Siegal, H. (1988) *Educating Reason: Rationality, Critical Thinking and Education,* Routledge, London.

Styles, M.M. & Moccia, P. (eds) (1993) *On Nursing: A Literary Celebration,* National League for Nursing, New York.

Wallace, D. (1996) Experiential learning and critical thinking in nursing. *Nursing Standard,* **10** (31), 43–7.

Acknowledgements

This chapter draws significantly on the following unpublished work:

Atkins S. & Murphy K. (1993) *Developing Skills for Profiling Learning.* An unpublished open learning package. Oxford Brookes University, Oxford.

Mackin J. (1997) *Reflections in the Mirror of Experience: Understanding the Ethical Dilemmas of Nursing Practice.* Unpublished doctoral dissertation and open learning package, Teachers College, Columbia University, New York.

My sincere thanks go to Kathy Murphy and Janet Mackin for their contributions.

Chapter 3
Assessment and Evaluation of Reflection

Introduction

Assessment and evaluation of reflection are emerging as crucial activities for generating evidence to confirm or refute the link between reflection and improvement in nursing practice. While reflection has become widely accepted in nurse education as an important method of developing practice with the potential to enhance the quality of health care delivery, there appears to be a lack of empirical evidence to support the belief that engaging in reflection actually changes practice or benefits patient care (Andrews *et al.*, 1998).

The purpose of this chapter is to explore some of the current issues surrounding assessment and evaluation of reflection. The prevailing issues are somewhat different from those examined in the first edition by Burns (1994). Indeed, in some aspects, such as the assessment of competence through reflective assignments, radical changes of opinion have occurred. These changes have been prompted by a number of factors; most notably the far-reaching changes that have recently occurred within the domains of health care and nurse education, together with issues that emerged from the assessment of reflection within early practice-led curricula in the late 1980s.

To explore fully the current issues pertaining to the assessment and evaluation of reflection, we will explore the following aspects within this chapter:

- the value of using reflection to assess learning within nurse education programmes
- the importance of context on curriculum, exploring the current climates of health care and education, and the way in which these environments have impacted upon the use of reflection within nurse education
- methods of assessment using reflection, highlighting practical examples of verbal and written assessments
- problems associated with assessing reflection

● issues concerning the evaluation of reflection and its impact on professional practice.

We conclude with some thoughts on what the future might hold in relation to assessment and evaluation of reflection within professional nursing practice.

The value of using reflection to assess learning

The use of reflection to assess learning within nurse education programmes has enormous potential, both for the individual student and for the profession. Incorporating reflection into the academic assessment process helps to formalise the use of reflection within academic curricula. It acknowledges the value of reflection for learning in professional practice and ensures that practice makes a significant contribution to the academic and practice outcomes of professional education. As nurse education has moved into the arena of higher education, the achievement of effective integration of reflection into academic processes has been challenging. In response to changing priorities within health care and professional nursing, practice-led curricula have developed which underpin current nurse education programmes. These programmes, both at pre- and post-registration level, incorporate an increased use of reflection in formal assessment strategies thus facilitating exploration and learning from practice. In this section we aim to explore the rationale for using reflection to assess learning within nurse education and to highlight some of the issues that surround the use of reflection in academic assessment.

The move to give equal priority to theory and clinical practice within assessment strategies has arisen as a result of changing perspectives on the nature and content of nurse education. Over the last decade, there has been growing recognition of the need to minimise the theory – practice gap, a factor identified as being negative to the development of competent practitioners (Gott 1984, Melia 1987). Simultaneously, there has been a growing acceptance of the need to develop practitioners who are 'fit for purpose', a phrase that Rushforth and Ireland (1997) suggest has become widely adopted for describing practitioners who have the knowledge, skills and attitudes to function independently within the present health care system. Thus, an emergent practitioner who is 'fit for purpose' is capable of undertaking the role that nurse education has prepared them for and responds effectively to challenges encountered within the reality of nursing practice. To ensure that practitioners have the opportunity to develop the skills and knowledge required for their professional lives, practice and analysis of practice must be at the centre of the curriculum (Bines & Watson 1992). Reflection can play a key part in this process.

We believe that, within a practice-led curriculum, strategies that facilitate learning from practice should be integrated at every level, including that of assessment. The use of reflection in the assessment of learning represents one way of bringing the complexities of practice and academic exploration closer together, helping to minimise the existence of a theory-practice gap. Such an approach also provides an appropriate mechanism for determining whether the outcome of developing a practitioner who is 'fit for purpose' has been achieved. Further more, we welcome the notion that within a practice-led curriculum, reflection and analysis of practice could contribute to the students' overall academic grade. By using reflection to assess learning, practice becomes integral to the academic assessment procedure and becomes valued equally alongside empirical knowledge sources.

The use of reflection encourages analysis of clinical practice; this, in turn, helps the practitioner to develop his or her knowledge and to acquire a deeper level of understanding about the complexities of nursing practice. Boud *et al.* (1985) suggest that this type of learning contributes to the development of clinical competence.

The literature displays a lack of consensus about what constitutes competence in clinical nursing practice. In relation to competency as described in this chapter we would subscribe to the definition offered by Butler (1978) cited in Chambers (1998): ' "the ability to meet or surpass prevailing standards of adequacy for a particular activity", implying that there is more than one level of competence and that one may be competent at any one activity whilst remaining incompetent at another.' (Chambers 1998, p. 202)

Marton & Saljo (1976) describe 'deep' approaches to learning as striving towards understanding, evaluating and relating knowledge to the students' own experience which, in itself promotes a motivation to learn. This emphasises the fact that clinical competence is not just about 'doing' and the development of technical skills, but that it incorporates knowledge and attitudinal components as well. We believe that these arguments highlight the potential of reflection in and on practice to contribute to the development of clinical competence. The use of reflection within academic assessments may also facilitate the development of higher levels of academic thinking, a deeper understanding of the nature of professional knowledge and the generation of new knowledge. Atkins & Murphy (1993) identify the skills required to be reflective as self assessment, description, critical analysis, synthesis and evaluation. These are the same skills required to achieve higher levels of academic thinking. (See

Sue Atkins' chapter, Chapter 2, for further work in this area.) We propose that by encouraging learners in the analysis of their own and others' practice that higher level academic skills may be encouraged. In addition, the process of analysing practice involves the exploration of both feelings and knowledge. This process can help to illuminate the different types of knowledge required for professional practice. This may include aesthetic, personal, moral and empirical knowledge (Carper 1978). Reflection on practice, therefore, may help the practitioner to gain a deeper understanding of the nature of knowledge within a practice profession. Moreover, the exploration of unique practice situations has the potential to generate new knowledge as learners are encouraged to identify alternatives to action, and devise solutions and strategies for managing situations more effectively in the future. We propose that this aspect of reflection has the potential to promote personal and professional growth and, thus, improvements in clinical practice.

To summarise, we believe that the use of reflection to assess learning within nurse education programmes has the potential to:

- draw on and value practice within the curriculum
- contribute to reducing the theory–practice gap
- promote the development of practitioners who are 'fit for purpose'
- contribute to the development of clinical competence
- encourage deep-level learning within the complex environment of nursing practice
- develop higher level academic skills, such as critical analysis, synthesis and evaluation
- promote personal and professional growth and, thus, improvements in clinical practice.

The changing climates of health care and education

Health care

Those who have had contact with the health care environment in recent years will have witnessed a considerable amount of change and it is generally recognised that this rapid pace of change is likely to continue in the foreseeable future. These changes have had a consequential impact upon the way in which nursing care is organised within the health service, resulting in:

- reduced numbers of permanent and qualified nursing staff, with an increase in non-permanent and unqualified health care staff requiring supervision

- increased numbers of patients requiring treatment (i.e. increased patient throughput or turnover in acute provider settings)
- more dependent patient population, due to higher levels of acuity, increased complexity of problems and shorter length of stays
- increased patient expectations in relation to quality of service delivery
- tighter focus on savings – targets often achieved through nursing staff vacancies or reduced support for professional development
- emphasis on quality improvement and clinical effectiveness
- low levels of staff morale
- increasing demand for newly qualified nurses who are skilled and able to perform their role fully at the point of qualification.

We recognise that these factors within the clinical environment have had considerable impact upon the availability of resources for facilitating student learning. Factors such as these have also contributed to changes within the pre-registration undergraduate nursing programme in Oxford, particularly in relation to the assessment of learning through academic assignments.

The strategy for the assessment of reflection within the original programme is described by Burns (1992, 1994) and examined further in the following section. This system relied heavily on the use of learning contracts and it was assumed that both the process and outcome of reflection (competence) could be assessed effectively through this one tool. Our experience of this integrated approach showed that students found it complex and difficult to master. In addition, mentors and service managers expressed concern about the intensity of resources required to support learners with this assessment framework. In practice modules, mentors were expected to contribute to the assessment process in numerous ways:

- assisting students to explore learning objectives, resources and strategies for achieving their objectives
- facilitating reflective discussions with learners to deepen their understanding of practice
- reading early drafts of students' reflective writing, providing feedback and initiating a dialogue about issues regarding practice situations reflected upon
- validating the achievement of competencies within the learning contract
- attending the student's final grading meeting and offering their opinion on the academic grade of the learning contract.

While the resource implications of the assessment strategy within the original undergraduate programme have been briefly acknowledged

(Burns 1994), this high level of mentor involvement has proved increasingly difficult to sustain within the current health care climate. In the revised pre-registration undergraduate programme, strategies used to assess learning are markedly less resource intensive, this is explored further on in the chapter.

Education

Similarly, nurse education has experienced its own challenges in recent years. Some key factors which have impacted upon education programmes in Oxford, and may have impacted elsewhere, are given here to illustrate this point:

- the drive to increase student numbers in response to the recruitment crisis (Royal College of Nursing 1996)
- emphasis on developing students who are 'fit for purpose' in response to health service demand, through more rigorous approaches to developing and assessing clinical competence
- moves in higher education to rationalise programmes by reducing number of modules and length of programmes and integrating modules/courses through shared-learning initiatives
- reduction of the trend towards over-assessment within nurse education programmes
- shift away from one-to-one practice based tutorials towards group teaching to free up resources
- continued concern for developing students who are also 'fit for the future' (Rushforth and Ireland 1997).

The current climate within nurse education is one of increasing student numbers but without a corresponding rise in the numbers of educational staff (Lowe & Kerr 1998). This is coupled with drives to increase student and mentor self reliance and to improve the effective use of resources through rationalisation at many levels. There appears to be a stronger emphasis on the achievement of competence, balanced with a continuing concern to develop students who will be able to respond to future developments in the health service.

In conclusion, the changing demands of health care and education in recent years have certainly had an impact on approaches used to assess and evaluate reflection within some of our courses. Key developments that have emerged as a result of these are:

- separation of the assessment of competence from the assessment of reflection

- development of a new method for the assessment of competence
- re-focusing the mentors' role on the assessment of clinical competence and coaching and away from assessment of academic ability
- emphasis on the facilitation of learning from practice, in group settings rather than in one-to-one tutorials
- use of a range of other reflective assessment tools in practice modules, such as critical incident analysis and reflective case studies, in addition to reflective learning contracts.

How can we assess reflection?

'How can we assess reflection?' is a key question that is, in the main, poorly answered in the literature. Discussion mainly focuses on the process of reflection, the skills needed for reflection and interpretation of the concept of reflection (Atkins & Murphy 1993, James & Clarke 1994). Much of the literature appears to ignore the issue of assessment and as Wong *et al.* (1995) note, this could be due to the lack of acceptable methods for assessing whether or not reflection takes place. There is the belief identified by some (Richardson 1995, Procter & Reed 1993) that any attempt to assess reflection contributes to reducing it. Procter and Reed (1993) note that the very act of assessing reflective activity can alter the students' way of thinking.

To set the scene, a brief background to the pre-registration undergraduate assessment strategy in Oxford will be given as this is where the most radical changes have occurred. Strategies for assessing reflection will be described and examples will be presented of techniques and methods utilised. An overview of the difficulties in assessing reflection will then be outlined.

Background to the assessment strategy in Oxford

When the nursing and midwifery pre-registration degree programme was first developed in Oxford, in 1989, reflective learning was a central component of the course and it was felt that the assessment strategy should reflect this. The work of Schön (1987), Boud *et al.* (1985), Benner (1984), Carper (1978) and Goodman (1984) had a major influence on the development of this undergraduate programme and also impacted on some of the post-qualifying and postgraduate courses.

With reflective learning as such a central component to the course, it was important to incorporate appropriate strategies for assessing reflection, which combined both theoretical and practice elements of the students' learning experience. Burns (1994) noted the increased importance attached to the relationships between nurse and patient and to patient-centred approaches to nursing care which warranted practitioners scrutinising their own values, beliefs and the context of care. She also recognised that the new curricular developments such as the introduction of Project 2000 emphasised the development of 'knowledgeable doers'. The conclusion was that in the unpredictable domain of nursing practice, it was not satisfactory to assess only outcomes of reflective learning but that the process should be assessed too.

Reflective learning contracts were felt to meet this need and were used extensively. However, as curricular developments progressed, other approaches have been developed which utilise reflective skills and so the range of assessment has broadened.

Reflective learning contracts

The advantages of using reflective learning contracts are clear, in that their use enables the integration of theory and practice. This type of coursework is student centred as the learning objectives would be based on the student's personal interests and around his or her own practice situations. The students would utilise the knowledge and experience of their mentors, link lecturers and lecturer practitioners (Lathlean 1992) together with an examination of literature to develop learning. The nature of practice could be analysed, feelings and values explored and the nature of knowledge and skills used could be identified. In addition, the need for new knowledge, skills or approaches could be examined.

The basic structure for the learning contracts is as follows:

- **Set objectives:** students develop specific practice-based learning objectives based on their own personal needs and interests, the expected course learning outcomes and the available learning opportunities in the placement area.
  For example:
    'To examine my role in detecting and reducing urinary tract infections in a ward environment.'
    'To explore the psychological impact of acute changes in health status on acute medical patients and the nurse's role in providing support'.
- **Identify resources and strategies:** this involves identifying what the student needs to do to achieve the given objective. It could include drawing on identified clinical expertise and observing or participating in certain activities within the practice area. This section of the learning contract also contains a list of references used in the evidence section of the text, these would be presented in full, using a recognised academic style of referencing.

Some students were quite creative in seeking out learning opportunities; for example: a student 'followed a urine specimen' from the ward to the laboratories to examine issues of specimen storage and its influence on the accuracy of results.

- **Evidence and reflection:** by reflecting on the experiences of themselves and others, students provide evidence that they have achieved the objective set. This is in the form of a narrative (see the chapters in this book containing exemplars) which encompasses all stages of the reflective cycle (Gibbs 1988) and provides evidence of personal learning. Students are encouraged to keep a reflective diary and to draw examples from this to utilise in their learning contract. In some learning contracts, the students are also required to demonstrate achievement of clinical competence within their reflective narrative.

- **Validation:** this section is for the mentor, link lecturer or lecturer practitioner to add comments and feedback. The best learning contracts are those which demonstrate dynamic development in response to these comments. For example: a student critically describes a negative encounter with a member of the multi-disciplinary team, the mentor asks the student to try and address the other person's perspective and she may also be able to give feedback on the skill with which the student handled the encounter. The student then develops the narrative to include these issues and possibly others stimulated by the mentor's feedback.

The assessment of this reflective evidence is carried out using a grading grid that allocates marks under the following headings:

- Identification of learning situations
- Description of situation, thoughts and feelings
- Analysis of feelings
- Analysis of knowledge
- Evidence of learning.

Utilising the grading criteria, students achieve a higher grade if their reflection addresses the relationship between principles and practice and incorporates political and ethical issues (Goodman 1984). A lower grade is achieved if the reflection is only descriptive and focuses purely on techniques needed to reach the desired objective. Therefore, critical analysis of the issues is graded higher than simple description.

There have been, however, some concerns about the dependence on this type of learning contract throughout the curriculum, within pre-registration preparation. This type of learning contract is still in use in our post-registration programmes where the experience and maturity of the students have enabled them to cope better with the reflective learning contract as described above.

In order to examine these concerns about the pre-registration programme a small pilot study was carried out which scrutinised reflective learning contracts (Schutz *et al.* 1996). Interviews with students and mentors were also carried out to gain their views. The students felt that the learning contract actually deflected their energy away from practice and cited the volume of writing as a particular concern.

The following is a summary of the conclusions from the study:

- The learning contract was considered unwieldy as it tried to do too much; assess competence, reflective and academic skills.
- The documentation of competency in learning contracts did not distinguish between exceptional or mediocre practice.
- The validation of competence was often occurring irrespective of the reflective evidence in the learning contract
- Although context was recognised in the writing of contracts the time spent on the process of writing removed students from experiencing practice.

As a response to this feedback and the impact of increased pressures in the clinical area, in the undergraduate pre-registration programme, the assessment of competence has been separated from the learning contract. The mentor's role has been restricted to assessing student competence and coaching and the academic assessment of reflective written work lies with university staff attached to the practice area. This change is currently being monitored and will be evaluated over time. It is hoped that such a change will free up the students to be reflective but not be overburdened by copious amounts of writing in an attempt to fit all the competencies they have met within the confines of a reflective learning contract.

Other assessment strategies

A number of strategies are available to assess reflection. This is a brief overview of some of these verbal and written approaches; reflective discussions, tutorial groups, and various means of assessing written reflection. It is hoped that as our assessment strategy develops in Oxford, more varied and creative approaches will continue to be developed.

As can be seen in Figure 3.1, the use of reflection continues to underpin the philosophy for practice and learning. Mentors are introduced to

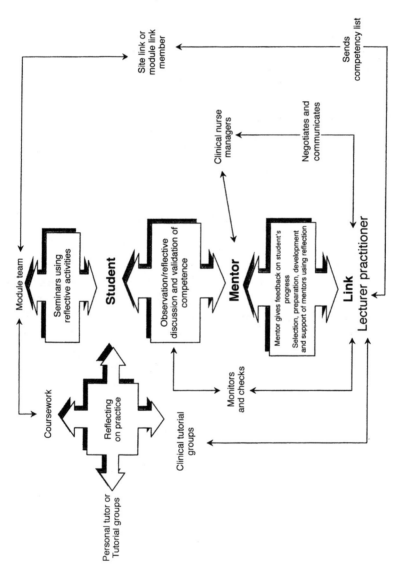

Fig. 3.1 Diagrammatic representation of the relationship between assessment of competence and reflection (in the current undergraduate pre-registration programme in Oxford) and its relationship with practice.

reflection during the mentor preparation day and there is a strong emphasis placed on the mentor, facilitating student learning using verbal reflection-on-practice to demonstrate both the knowledge and attitude that the student has to underpin his or her practice skills. Verbal reflection is also used as a strategy for learning in seminar and tutorial groups and as explained feeds into the assessment strategy.

Verbal assessment strategies

Reflective discussions between mentor and student

The preparation of mentors includes an introduction to the concept of reflection and to Johns' (1995) framework for structured reflection. Mentors may also be familiar with the concept of reflection from their own study, through clinical supervision or from the use of reflective strategies used in the clinical area.

These practice mentors work alongside students in their day-to-day practice experience. During these encounters the mentors and the student will try and find time to reflect on their experiences and learning. These reflective encounters may not happen every day, but depend on such factors as workload, the quality of the relationship and the commitment of both the mentor and the student (see Brigid Reid's chapter, Chapter 4, on mentoring). This interaction may involve the mentor 'making explicit' her thought processes, decision making and feelings. Likewise the student may be challenged to examine his or her own beliefs and values relating to a situation or encounter.

> As an example: an inexperienced student was asked by her mentor to feed a patient who had recently had a stroke. The student felt very uncomfortable, as she had never fed anyone before. At the end of the shift the student reflected on the situation and realised she needed further support. She spent some time asking the mentor specific questions about her own experiences and throughout this process realised she needed to find out more about the effect of a stroke on the patient's ability to eat. At the suggestion of her mentor, she also tried to imagine what it was like to be in the patient's position and think about how she could involve the family in assessing the patient's needs. Her mentor also reflected on what her student had experienced and realised that she could have better prepared the student for the task, she thought seriously about her own accountability for the patient's safety. The student also realised through her reflections that she also has a responsibility to ask for more information prior to undertaking an unfamiliar activity.

These kinds of reflective encounters may not always be assessed directly, but they often feed into the assessment process. One of the mentor's responsibilities is to verify by signing that the student has achieved competence in given areas. These competency statements include attitude and knowledge as well as skill. Reflective discussions such as the one outlined above contribute to providing evidence to the mentor regarding the achievement of these elements, in this instance, the competencies relating to nutrition and to comfort. The students will also be developing their thinking and self awareness in the context of real practice and so this practice-related knowledge may also feed into written assessments.

Tutorials

Individual and group tutorials are a regular occurrence within our programmes in Oxford. However, as resources tighten, and because of demographic and political changes, there has been a need to reduce to a minimum the routine 'labour intensive' one-to-one tutorials with our students. In the past, this was where considerable reflective activity took place. Subsequently there has been the increased development of group tutorials.

Throughout the diverse range of programmes in the School of Health Care, group tutorials have been used sporadically. The development of a new pre-registration undergraduate 3-year nursing and midwifery programme has provided an opportunity to formalise the development of these groups, specifically those facilitated by the professional tutor. The aim of these group tutorials is to introduce the students to the notion of reflection early on in the programme. Rather than expect students to engage in the more advanced skills of reflection, we gradually introduce the development of skills such as self awareness, detailed description and critical analysis.

Heath (1998) comments that new students are often overwhelmed by the plethora of information and experiences and it is difficult for them to reflect. Although this gently paced introduction to reflection is a relatively new approach, the initial feedback from students and staff is positive. Students comment that it is useful to share experiences and for the tutorial leader it is a good opportunity to promote reflection and the analysis of practice situations.

> For example, in a tutorial group students were discussing what they had done on their first few shifts in practice. One student was very disappointed that she had not done anything exciting, but had spent some time making beds. I asked the student how she made the bed and she described the process clearly. I then asked her why she had done it in that way. She answered that she had done it that way because her mentor had shown her. The tutorial group were then asked about their own experiences and we

then developed the discussion to include all the factors that would influence the way we made a bed such as infection control issues, timing of bed-making, patient comfort issues, ritualistic practice and pressure sore risks. We also examined the students' beliefs and values relating to what was important in nursing.

This simple example illustrates how with facilitation, a situation that at the time was not a learning experience for the student was developed and shared. By promoting the process of reflection in a group environment the students will hopefully develop skills that will enable them to give rationale for their care decisions. These skills will then enable them articulate achievement of the knowledge, skill and attitude needed for the validation of competence by the mentor, which is one aspect of the assessment of practice. It is also hoped that these activities will promote self awareness and critical thinking and that the analysis of practice at a deeper level will then feed into their written coursework, which is then formally assessed.

Reflective group tutorials can also be facilitated by seminar leaders, or in the placement areas by the link lecturer or lecturer practitioner. Individual tutorials are still available for the discussion of personal issues or where the student needs extra support.

As an example, in a seminar with the aim of introducing students to the 'patient's experience of health care', the students were asked to reflect on their own encounters with health care and to think about how it felt for them. They were asked to identify the negative and positive factors that impacted on the situation and what could have been done differently to improve the experience for themselves. This personal reflection then fed into discussion around the theoretical perspective of holism and its implications for the students' own future practice.

Although reflective incidents such as the two described above do not feed directly into the formal assessment process, they give some insight into the students' progression and learning. They may also contribute to removing blocks to students' future learning caused by anxiety or misunderstandings.

The facilitators of group tutorials need to ensure that students who are reluctant to contribute to the group do not get neglected and are enabled to engage in these reflective activities. A good knowledge of the workings of groups and well-developed group facilitation skills are imperative in this role. There may be some benefit in mixing students from different years in the same tutorial groups. Heath (1998) suggests that this may enhance development of reflective skills. However, such a strategy would need careful assessment and evaluation.

Written assessment strategies

For written work, there are a number of activities that utilise reflection. Some of these are outlined below. Perry (1997) for example, notes that in the case of critical incident analysis, the writing reveals detailed insight into the working lives of nurses. It is possible to utilise both an academic and reflective style of writing in such assignments by giving the students a clear structure to work from. Reflective writing is much easier for the students when it is written in the first person, to not recognise the notion of 'self' in an arena that is reflexive is incongruent.

Wong *et al.* (1995) recognised that student writing may not be indicative of reflective ability; although they attempted to test this with a verbal interview, numbers in the study were relatively small and so the conclusions may need further testing. This is certainly an area that warrants further research.

Reflective diaries

Using reflective diaries or journal keeping as it is sometimes known, is a good starting point for reflective writing. Keeping a diary preserves time and space for reflective activity (Wong *et al.* 1995). By writing about our practice experience, we can more readily articulate the subtleties of what we do, this is a valuable skill as the nursing profession strives to define itself. Derbyshire (1991) introduces a series of narrative writings called 'Nursing reflections' by stating that when reflective writing is combined with interpretation it can encourage deeper understanding and will sometimes result in a change of perspective for the individual.

The use of reflective diaries is in the main felt to be beneficial. Durgahee (1997) notes a variety of benefits including promoting the instigation of purposeful observation, scrutiny of the nurses role, progression of intellectual focusing of practice issues, more questioning, increased confidence and the development of critical thinking. Some nurses find the process of writing a cathartic experience that helps them to personally 'work through' problems or difficult situations.

Diaries are usually owned by the individual and are private. Difficulties can arise if the reflection highlights poor practice or even disciplinary issues (Burns 1994). This can be avoided if the ownership of the diaries clearly lies with the student. There may be situations where issues of poor practice that have been highlighted need to be tactfully fed back to the practice area.

The idea of assessing reflective diaries is problematic. It is crucial therefore that students are aware that their writings will be assessed from the outset. Richardson & Maltby (1995) utilised a study and framework by Powell (1989) for the measurement of reflectivity from reflective diaries and focus group interviews. They noted that some students found the assessment of their diaries to be a barrier. They also found, as Powell did, that the majority of students did not use the higher levels of reflection. These higher levels are those that result in critical enquiry and problem solving.

If reflective diaries are used at all for assessment purposes, it may be beneficial to keep the assessment simple. Wong *et al.* (1995) carried out a small study examining reflection from student journal writings. They graded the students into one of three categories: non-reflector, reflector and critical reflector. Initial results from this study appear positive, although again the numbers involved were small.

In Oxford, the approach used is that student diaries are kept private. The students can select extracts that they wish to share for discussion in tutorial groups or with their mentor. They also may include some of the reflective elements in their writing of reflective essays or incident analysis. So this reflection may become assessed as part of the process of validating competence or grading of academic coursework.

Critical incident analysis

The notion of critical incident analysis is not new, it was used by pilots who analysed flying missions with the intent of improving their performance (Flanagan, 1954). Since then Smith & Russell (1991) and more recently Norman *et al.* (1992) and Perry (1997) have described it as an appropriate strategy in nurse education.

Critical incident analysis enables the students to utilise an incident from practice, reflect upon it and analyse it. The incident can be any incident that had an impact, positive or negative (Smith & Russell 1991). It can be a distinct incident with a beginning and end, or it may arise from identifying issues within an incident (Norman *et al.* 1992).

Perry (1997) acknowledges that analysis of an incident may provide a framework for 'reflection-on-action'. Smith & Russell (1991) provide useful guidance for students in the appendix of their paper. An example of a framework is given below:

(1) Give a concise description of the incident (which relates to the learning outcomes).
(2) Outline the rationale for choice of incident and its significance and relevance to you.
(3) Identify pertinent issues related to the incident.
(4) Reflect on and analyse the key issues focusing on:
     your own involvement, feelings and decision making

the involvement and role of others
identification of any dilemmas or ethical elements
the rationale for action, drawing on relevant theory
evaluation of the situation and the implications for practice and
personal learning.

(5)   Conclusion.

This method can be useful in assessing the student's ability to recognise the context of a situation and to promote the integration of the theoretical and the practical. Verbal structured analysis of incidents is also useful in the reflective discussion arena described previously.

Reflective essays

The essay as an assessment tool is well recognised. Such well developed techniques can be modified to assess reflective learning. These reflective essays are written using the same basic structure as a standard essay with an introduction, main body and conclusion. The idea being that by using reflection in the essay, the students' own involvement in the situation is explicit and their own experience of practice issues can be talked about. An example title might be:

Write an essay entitled:

Reflection upon and analysis of the nurse's role in discharge planning in a multi-professional environment

Here marks would still be awarded for academic style and structure, but the reflective element would be added to the generic grading criteria. For an example see Figure 3.2.

Case studies

In a case study, the student can examine the care delivered in a structured way, perhaps using a nursing model or framework.

For example:

Choose one aspect of care, explore the evidence-base for practice and critically analyse the nursing management for that aspect of care. Reflect on how the nursing management of the problem could have been improved.

This type of assignment clearly enables the student to make the connections with 'real' practice and the available theory. The student could look at his or her own assessment, planning and delivery of care

Criteria	Fail	Range from C to B+ ⇐ B ⇒	A
Analysis of thoughts and feelings	Does not demonstrate self awareness in written work	Consistently identifies feelings of both self and others	Consistently demonstrates insight into the situation. Evidence that analysis of feelings has informed practice
Description of the situation	Relevance of description unclear, lacks cohesion, organisation and clarity	Comprehensive, less able to discriminate relevant and irrelevant detail. Coherent, logical organisation	Consistently captures the essence of the situation. Succinct description of relevant features. Fluent expression, lively stimulating style
Evidence of personal and professional developments and implications for practice	Lacks evidence of personal learning or indication of learning for future practice. No attempt to offer solutions to identified problems and no alternatives to action taken	Good account of personal learning with some indication of its value to practice. Offers solutions to identified problem, alternatives to action taken are given, identifying a plan for implementation	Evaluates personal learning and clearly relates this to future practice. Offers solutions to identified problems and alternatives to action taken, with creative strategies for implementation

Fig. 3.2 Examples of additional 'reflective' elements added to the generic grading assessment criteria (School of Health Care, Oxford Brookes University).

and evaluate its effectiveness. This sort of exercise will equip students with a clear rationale for their care decisions that may prove useful to them in their professional lives.

Assessment criteria

Many of our programmes use a generic assessment criteria which includes; critical analysis of theory and literature, use of literature, presentation, structure and conclusions. All these criteria are graded from 'A' grade to fail accordingly. In an assignment that incorporates a reflective element, additional components may be added to the generic grid that relates to the development of the skills of reflection such as self awareness, analysis and synthesis (see Figure 3.2).

Although levels of reflection are widely mentioned in the literature in relation to depth or progression, the association of these levels with assessment has not been further examined in great detail. It does appear that in many of these descriptors of 'reflective progression', higher-level reflection includes broader issues, application to practice or perspective transformation.

Mezirow (1981) generated seven levels of reflection that are considered to be highly theoretical and are widely quoted. Powell (1989) and Coutts-Jarman (1993) adapted these to the practical considerations of nursing. Powell's adaptation of Mezirow's framework clearly shows the developing stages from simple description or observation, to evaluation and judgement to exploring concepts resulting in altered action or perspective. Powell concludes from her study that in the main, nurses used the lower levels of reflection, the exception being those in autonomous roles such as nurse practitioners.

Similar to Goodman's (1984) levels utilised in Oxford's reflective learning contract assessment, Smith and Hatton (1993, in Johns & Freshwater 1998) describe three levels which graduate from the descriptive, through the dialogic stage and on to critical. Conversely, Richardson (1995) sees reflective thought processes not as linear, hierarchical processes of thinking, but as multi-faceted which may be entered and exited. If we use levels to assess, then we need to determine each student's starting point, which may be difficult to achieve as until the reflective process is underway, the student or assessor may not realise where the starting point is.

There is still considerable work to be done on grading criteria for assessing reflection. There is perhaps scope to explore in greater depth the levels of reflection particularly relating to assessment with the hope of devising a valid and reliable tool. Until validated frameworks or tools are available then it is worth being aware that some of these criteria are untested.

Reflective processes and outcomes are still such intangibles, that attempting to assess them opens up a minefield of difficulties. The confusion relating to assessment strategies is not surprising, as there are wide interpretations of the notion and practical application of reflection. There is also the apparent overlap of terms such as reflection, reflective practice and reflective learning and to some extent some commonalties with concepts such as critical thinking and critical analysis. Many of the skills such as self awareness, analysis and 'finding meaning' are common to more than one of these concepts. Some of the expected outcomes are common such as development of practice and of the individual. Until we have greater clarity in the expected outcomes of reflection, it will remain difficult to assess them and so make the connection as to how the process of reflection is helping achieve the outcomes.

Although some of these problems in assessing reflection have been discussed earlier in the chapter, a summary is given in Figure 3.3.

The idea of assessing reflection is fraught with potential problems relating to confusions, current climates and practical realities. The solution may lie in a flexible approach enabling some freedom of reflection for the student, yet some standardisation for assessment purposes.

Problems with assessing reflection	Authors who have written on this area
Lack of available tools	Wong *et al.* 1995
Overlap of terms such as reflective practice, reflective learning, critical thinking and critical analysis	Daly 1998
What should be assessed, process or outcome?	Mountford & Rogers 1996, Burns 1994
What are the outcomes? Can they be distinguished from other factors? What are the stages of the process?	James & Clark 1994, Lowe & Kerr 1998, Mezirow
Reflection is a complex activity and is especially difficult for new students	Heath 1998
Reflective activities will be undermined if assessed	Richardson 1995
Students will not reflect honestly if assessed	Richardson 1995
Lack of validation of reflection/risk of bias or inaccuracy	Saylor 1990, Andrews *et al.* 1998, James & Clark 1994, Fitzgerald 1994
Lack of skill/bias of facilitators of reflection	Andrews *et al.* 1998, Durgahee 1998
Health care is product rather than process orientated (political and financial pressures)	Richardson 1995
Reflection is a time consuming activity	Pierson 1998
Reflection draws on tacit knowledge which may be difficult to articulate	Meerabeau 1992

Fig. 3.3 Problems with assessing reflection.

The implications for staff

As within any educational programme the university staff and mentors themselves have varied ability and skill to facilitate reflection and do so utilising different frameworks or structures. Durgahee (1998) recognises this, and coins the phrases 'guide on the side' as opposed to 'sage on the stage' to distinguish between facilitative and controlling teaching strategies. There is an obvious potential benefit for utilising a clinical supervision framework to enable staff to explore their own progression in developing reflective skills. It may be of benefit to provide supervision or at the very least some training for staff new to the role.

The question of validity causes concern in relation to assessment. Students may be articulate and 'tell us what we want to hear', they may present a different account to one that is too painful for them to recall. The inaccuracy may not be purposeful; perhaps the student did not grasp the context or understand the complexities of a situation. Andrews *et al* (1998) assert that the supervisor must accept the honesty and validity of the reflection yet they recognise that this is a valid approach only when the process is considered the important element. If the reflection is verbal then perhaps the skilled facilitator can validate the experience, but a particular difficulty arises in written assessments.

The detailed analysis of student writing to identify the levels of reflection, or the transcribing of student interviews is feasible in the research domain, but in environments where workloads are high a simpler way of assessing reflection is required. This poses yet another area of conflict and difficulty. To simplify assessment criteria opens it to wider interpretation and misuse, yet to detail it results in it being unwieldy.

Evaluation of reflection

As reflection becomes integrated within nurse education, it is increasingly important to demonstrate the benefits of reflection on professional practice and health care delivery. We propose that it is only through effective evaluation that the impact of reflection on professional practice can be accurately measured.

It is argued that all educational activity demands evaluation (Herbener & Watson 1992). With the growing use of reflection within pre- and post-registration nurse education programmes during the 1990s, evaluation of such approaches must now be a priority. While reflection is perceived to play a key role in the development of effective practitioners, there is a lack of empirical evidence to support the belief that engaging in reflection actually changes practice or benefits patient care (Andrews *et al.* 1998). This highlights the need for evaluation strategies which focus specifically on the link between educational programmes and clinical effectiveness (Jordan 1988). (See Nettie Dearmun's and Brigid Reid's chapters, Chapters 8 and 4, within this book for their research in this area.)

Improvement in practice must be the ultimate aim of using reflection within any nurse education programme. We suggest that, to evaluate the use of reflection effectively, the focus must be on the learner's own development in practice and the impact that this has had on patient care. The question is how can a key outcome of reflection, that is the student's development in practice as a result of a reflective education programme, be measured? While reflective assignments as part of an assessment strategy could contribute to the evaluation strategy, this alone is unlikely to be sufficient. Writing about practice and how it has or will improve as a result of the reflective process may not equate to the amount of progress actually achieved by the individual. We also recognise that measuring an individual's development in practice as a direct result of reflection is fraught with difficulties, as so many other variables may be influential in this outcome.

As a first step, we suggest that it is valuable to consider potential outcomes of reflection, as this helps to illuminate potential evaluation criteria. Boud *et al.* (1985) suggest that the outcomes of reflection may be both cognitive and affective in nature. They provide a comprehensive list of outcomes of reflection that they summarise in four key points:

(1) New perspectives on experience
(2) Change in behaviour
(3) Readiness for application
(4) Commitment to action.

Reflective learning, then, may involve students changing their perspective on practice as a result of experience. It may also lead to changes in attitudes, values and behaviour. The learner should demonstrate motivation to apply new knowledge and skills learned and should be committed to utilising these in practice. There may also be a deepening of understanding of a student's own learning style and needs, and a positive attitude towards further learning. The work of Boud *et al.* (1985) implies that a change in the way practitioners think and practice are likely outcomes of reflective processes. We are aware, however, that measurement of the outcomes of reflection may not be a straightforward activity. Boud *et al.* (1985) recognise that some of these outcomes are intangible and may not be easily demonstrated or observed in practice.

Others take time to develop and may only be evident some time after the end of an education programme. Thus, questions emerge about the most effective strategy for accurately measuring the outcomes of reflection.

While the issue of evaluation of reflection within the literature is recognised, a limited number of studies have been conducted in this area to date. Thus, as a vehicle for raising some prevailing issues concerning the evaluation of reflection, we will use the example of a post-registration course entitled 'Principles in Acute Medical Nursing'. This is a practice-based course that is run collaboratively between the Oxford Radcliffe Hospitals NHS Trust and Oxford Brookes University. The strategies used within this course to assess and evaluate progress in practice and knowledge and the impact of these on patient care are:

- two academic assignments, including a critical incident analysis and a reflective case study
- a base line self assessment of practice undertaken in relation to a number of predetermined practice learning outcomes, which is validated by a practice mentor
- a written summary of evidence of achievement in relation to practice learning outcomes, which is validated by the mentor and reviewed by the academic supervisor
- a brief summary of progress in relation to the practice learning outcomes provided by the mentor
- evaluation questionnaires which are distributed to the student, mentor and ward manager three months after the completion of the course.

The main focus of the evaluation questionnaires is the degree of change in the student's practice since undertaking the course and the extent to which new knowledge and skills have been applied in practice. The questions are based around the following criteria and respondents are asked to provide an illustrative example for each item:

- development of knowledge
- development of skill
- development/change in attitude
- sharing of new knowledge/participation in educational activities
- participation in clinical development initiatives.

We recognise that this approach relies fairly heavily on individual perceptions concerning the learner's development in practice, and that perceptions are not always an accurate way of measuring actual progress achieved. However, the incorporation of illustrative examples does go some way towards introducing a degree of objectivity and a means of gathering evidence concerning the nature of the change in practice. We also acknowledge that the perspectives and outcomes of consumers are not incorporated into the course evaluation strategy at present. Andrews *et al.* (1998) state that patient outcomes should be measured to determine if the benefits of reflection are transmitted to patients and that without this it is difficult to assert that reflection influences patient care. Durgahee (1998) further suggests that patient perceptions of reflective practitioners should be included in any further evaluation of reflective practice. We are aware, however, that there are many difficulties associated with consumer feedback strategies and the development of valid and reliable methods for eliciting such information is inherently problematic. However, we propose that this must be highlighted as an area for further debate and research in the near future.

The need to evaluate the impact of reflection on practice and the delivery of health care is paramount, although we also recognise that this process is highly complex in nature. Research studies in this area are limited, although examples of evaluation of reflection do exist in practice and this information could be usefully shared among nurse educationalists and managers. The issue of evaluation of reflection has only just begun to be explored and it presents a considerable challenge for the future. We believe that the issues which require further consideration in relation to the evaluation of reflection are:

- the identification of strategies for pinpointing development in practice as a result of reflection rather than other influential variables
- the identification of methods which identify actual changes in practice as opposed to perceptions of changes in practice
- whether patient outcomes and perspectives could be incorporated into evaluation strategies and how this might be achieved most effectively
- the need for longitudinal studies to monitor long-term effects and benefits of reflection on individual practitioners and their practice.

Conclusion

Throughout this chapter the context of health care education has been recognised. The climate of both health care delivery and professional education is in a state of rapid change and there is increasing pressure to deliver cost effective and high quality services. It has been suggested that reflection is a process that can contribute to developing nurses who meet these current and future demands by producing practitioners whose theoretical knowledge is grounded in practice and who have the self awareness and skills to become life long learners. The value of using reflection in assessment has been identified, but these benefits have not been proven yet and there is a need for larger-scale research to evaluate the effectiveness of the process and also to ascertain the outcomes.

Various strategies, both verbal and written for utilising reflection in assessment have been highlighted and the potential problems outlined. We believe that reflection is a valid means of learning. However, to assess and evaluate such a complex area is difficult, but is important to do so, as the benefits to the individual student and to practice need to be made explicit.

There is a definite place for reflection in assessment and evaluation in the future and some issues for future consideration are outlined here:

- The value of practice needs to be recognised in assessment strategies and reflection is an effective medium for this.
- Creative, realistic assessment strategies that utilise reflective processes need to be developed and shared.
- Reflective approaches need to be sustained in the current pressured health care and education climates.
- The relationship between perceptions expressed in verbal and written reflection and the impact on actual practice needs further investigation. Outcomes of reflection for the student, the patient and the profession need to be further identified and evaluated.
- Collaborative, large-scale research is needed to evaluate the benefits of reflection.

References

Andrews, M., Gidman, J. & Humphreys, A. (1998) Reflection: does it enhance professional nursing practice? *British Journal of Nursing*, **7** (7), 413–17.

Atkins, S. & Murphy, K. (1993) Reflection: a review of the literature. *Journal of Advanced Nursing*, **18**, 1188–92.

Benner, P. (1984) *From Novice to Expert: Excellence and Power in Clinical Nursing Practice*. Addison-Wesley, Menlo Park, California.

Bines, H. & Watson, D. (1992) *Developing Professional Education*, Society for Research into Higher Education and Open University Press, Buckingham.

Boud, D., Keogh, R. & Walker, (eds) (1985) *Reflection: Turning Experience into Learning*, Kogan Page Ltd, London.

Burns, S. (1992) Grading practice, *Nursing Times*, **88** (1), 40–42.

Burns, S. (1994) *Assessing reflective learning*. In Palmer, A., Burns, S. & Bulman, C. *Reflective Practice in Nursing; The Growth of the Professional Practitioner*, Blackwell Scientific Publications. Oxford.

Carper, B. (1978) Fundamental patterns of knowing in nursing. *Advances in Nursing Science*, **1** (v), 13–33.

Chambers, M.A. (1998) Some issues in the assessment of clinical practice: a review of the literature. *Journal of Clinical Nursing*, **7**, 201–208.

Coutts-Jarman, J. (1993). Using reflection and experience in nurse education. *British Journal of Nursing*, **2** (1), 77–80.

Daly, W. (1998) Critical thinking as an outcome of nursing education, what is it? Why is it important to nursing practice? *Journal of Advanced Nursing*, **28**, 323–31.

Derbyshire, P. (1991) Nursing reflections. *Nursing Times*, **87** (36), 27–8.

Durgahee, T. (1996) Promoting reflection in post-graduate nursing: a theoretical model. *Nurse Education Today*, **16** (6), 419–26.

Durgahee, T. (1997) Reflective practice: nursing ethics through story telling. *Nursing Ethics*, **4** (2), 135–46.

Durgahee, T. (1998) Facilitating reflection: from a sage on the stage to a guide on the side. *Nurse Education Today*, **18**, 158–64.

Fitzgerald, M. (1994) *Theories of reflection for learning.* In Palmer, A., Burns, S. & Bulman, C. *Reflective Practice in Nursing; The Growth of the Professional Practitioner*, Blackwell Science, Oxford.

Flanagan, J.C. (1954) The critical incident technique. *Psychological Bulletin*, **51** 327–58.

Gibbs, G. (1988) *Learning by Doing. A Guide to Teaching and Learning Methods*, Further Education Unit, Oxford Polytechnic, Oxford.

Goodman, J. (1984) Reflection and teacher education: a case study and theoretical analysis. *Interchange*, **15**, 9–25.

Gott, M. (1984) *Learning Nursing*, Royal College of Nursing, London.

Heath, H. (1998). Reflection and patterns of knowing in nursing. *Journal of Advanced Nursing*, **27**, 1054–9.

Herbener, D. & Watson, J. (1992) Models for evaluating nursing education programs. *Nursing Outlook*, **40** (1), 27–32.

James, C. & Clarke, B. (1994) Reflective practice in nursing: issues and implications for nurse education. *Nurse Education Today*, **14**, 82–90.

Johns, C. (1995) Framing learning through reflection within Carper's Fundamental Ways of Knowing in Nursing. *Journal of Advanced Nursing*, **22**, 226–34.

Jordan, S. (1998) From classroom theory to clinical practice: evaluating the impact of a post-registration course. *Nurse Education Today*, **18**, 293–302.

Lowe, P. B. & Kerr, C. M. (1998) Learning by reflection: the effect on educational Outcomes. *Journal of Advanced Nursing*, **27**, 1030–33.

Lathlean, J. (1992) The contribution of lecturer practitioners to theory and practice in nursing. *Journal of Clinical Nursing*, **1**, 237–42.

Marton, F. & Saljo, R. (1976) On qualitative differences in learning 1, Outcome and process. *British Journal of Educational Psychology*, **46**, 4–11.

Melia, K. (1987) *Learning and Working – The Occupational Socialisation of Nurses*, Tavistock. London.

Meerabeau, L. (1992) Tacit nursing knowledge: an untapped resource or methodological headache. *Journal of Advanced Nursing*, **17**, 108–12.

Mezirow, J. (1981) A critical theory for adult learning and education. *Adult Education*, **32** (1), 3–24.

Mountford, B. & Rogers, L.(1996) Using individual and group reflection in and on assessment as a tool for effective learning. *Journal of Advanced Nursing*, **24**, 1127–34.

Norman, I., Redfern, S., Tomalin, D. & Oliver, S. (1992) Developing Flanagan's critical incident technique to elicit indicators of high and low quality nursing care from patients and their nurses. *Journal of Advanced Nursing*, **17**, 590–600.

Perry, L. (1997) Critical incidents, crucial issues: insights into the working lives of registered nurses. *Journal of Clinical Nursing*, **6**, 131–7.

Pierson W. (1998) Reflection and nurse education. *Journal of Advanced Nursing*, **27**, 165–70.

Powell, J. (1989) The reflective practitioner in nursing. *Journal of Advanced Nursing*, **14**, 824–32.

Procter, S. & Reed, J. (1993). Assessment of reflection. In Reed, J. & Procter, S. (1993) *Nurse Education. A reflective approach*, Edward Arnold, London.

Richardson, G. & Maltby, H. (1995) Reflection on practice: enhancing student learning. *Journal of Advanced Nursing*, **22**, 235–42.

Richardson, R. (1995) Humpty Dumpty: reflection and reflective nursing practice. *Journal of Advanced Nursing*, **21**, 1044–50.

Royal College of Nursing (1996) 'On the Edge', RCN Annual Congress, 23 April, Bournemouth.

Rushforth, H. & Ireland, L. (1997) Fit for whose purpose? The contextual forces underpinning the provision of nurse education in the UK. *Nurse Education Today*, **17**, 437–41.

Saylor, C.R. (1990) Reflection and professional education: art, science and competency, *Nurse Educator*, **15** (2), 8–11.

Schön, D.A. (1987) *Educating the Reflective Practitioner*, Jossey Bass, San Francisco.

Schutz, S., Bulman, C. & Salussolia, M. (1996) The learning contract as a tool for documenting competence. *Teaching News*, (Oxford Brookes University Publication) **43**, 17–18.

Smith, D. & Hatton, N. (1993) *Critical reflection on action in professional education*. 5th National Practicum Conference. February 1993. Macquarie University, Sydney. In Johns, C. & Freshwater, D. (1998) *Transforming Nursing through reflective practice*, Blackwell Science, Oxford.

Smith, A. & Russell, J. (1991) Using critical incidents in nurse education. *Nurse Education Today*, **11** (4), 284–91.

Wong, F., Kember, D., Chung, L & Yan, L. (1995) Assessing the level of student reflection from reflective journals. *Journal of Advanced Nursing*, **22**, 48–57.

Chapter 4
The Role of the Mentor to Aid Reflective Practice

Introduction

Having a mentor can make a difference to learning. I made this claim in my original chapter (first edition) and I am now in a position to further endorse it from the benefit of additional experience and research. In 1994 I wrote directly from the personal perspective of being a mentor, offering my experiences of using strategies to promote and manage reflection with undergraduate nursing students. Since then I have undertaken education and practice roles and most recently that of researcher, exploring how competence is assessed in undergraduate nursing students. In these roles the skills of reflecting and promoting reflection in others have been essential. In revisiting my original chapter many of my thoughts have remained the foundation of my current thinking. I believe that the skill of reflection is vital to the development of practice and that there are active strategies that can assist in the development of such skills. This view was endorsed by the findings of my research (Reid 1997), which highlighted the role of the mentor in the education of undergraduate nursing students.

This chapter therefore is informed from a range of practice perspectives integrating and challenging theory as appropriate. Throughout I retain my belief that offering a flexible and unique balance between strategies of challenge and support for practitioners (be they undergraduate nursing students or post-registration staff) is central to being a mentor. Such a skill is complex and involves a high degree of self awareness. Because of this the needs of the role itself also require consideration if it is to be developed and sustained.

The reflective mentor

In supporting a learner to develop and manage reflection, the mentor must have a grasp not only of clinical practice but also of reflection. Reflection is a process of reviewing an experience of practice in order to describe, analyse, evaluate and so inform learning about practice. In contrast to the vision of quiet contemplation that the word used to create for me there is an active element to reflection. The activity which occurs in reflection involves moving beyond the experience as illustrated by the reflective cycle (Gibbs 1988) see Figure 4.2. The starting point for the cycle occurs when one questions why an outcome has occurred (Jarvis 1992). Such a question may arise from a feeling of discomfort (Boyd & Fales 1983), or from a dramatic event. From personal experience it is often the latter that novice students focus on. However it is important to recognise that we need to examine when we feel we have been effective and those activities which we take for granted to avoid habitualising our practice (Berger & Luckmann 1967).

As a mentor who is also a practitioner there is an issue of consciousness of self effect. My own use of reflection to learn from, inform and transform my practice has proved valuable in this respect. However I have learnt not to assume this is so for other practitioners. Powell (1989) wrote of how the practitioners in her small study had little insight into their actions; they did have knowledge informing them, but could not access or articulate it. Indeed the ability to articulate one's insight appears to be a skill that requires further development for all practitioners (Reid 1997). My understanding is that Powell's practitioners were previously unexposed to an atmosphere where reflection was promoted or indeed prevalent within nursing at that time. Reflecting upon my own development of reflection, environmental factors such as my colleagues' views have had an important role. Therefore development of reflective skills should not be considered as an 'add on' or isolated to key individuals, rather as a cultural issue for practice areas.

Using reflection can access our 'theories in use' (Powell 1989), so enabling others to learn. In this way, the risk of taking practice for granted has the potential to be reduced. For example, examine a departure from an unconscious routine in response to an individual's need. Often insight can be gained as to what influenced the action. Thus what we do; our 'artistry' (Schön, 1985), can be explored and shared. In recognising the role of reflection in this, its skill is relevant for both the learner and mentor.

In theory it may be possible to promote reflection without insight into the process but I suspect, from personal experience, to promote it you need to have used it. After I had been attempting to reflect, by keeping a diary for over a year, a chance conversation revealed to me that for the first time I was talking to someone who advocated reflection and actually practised it themselves! That a mentor should find some way of developing their reflective thinking is therefore, I believe, conducive to the process. I felt that my skills enabled me to be a credible and insightful role model, less threatened by reflective questioning and in a better position to be an effective validator of the students' contracts.

Strategies to promote reflection

Nurse education has increasingly relied upon ideas of adult education (Burnard 1990), the focus being on learning from experience and the ethos of self direction and responsibility on the part of the student. Reflection is more than describing experience, indeed in referring to the work of Nevitt Sandford on self reflection, Daloz asserted that it is:

> 'only by bringing our changes into conscious awareness that we can be assured they will stay put'.

> (Daloz 1986, p. 213)

It is in the involvement of guiding students through such transitions that Daloz feels mentors are vital. This is similar to Schön's (1985) concept of a 'coach'. Burnard (1990) however has doubts about such a close relationship, given the aims of adult education. He argues that rather than encouraging autonomy the mentor is more likely to foster dependence and conformity. It is the recognition of such a danger, and an awareness that adults often vary in their individual learning styles, that influence my consideration of strategies that mentors can use.

The work of Daloz (1986) on what it is that mentors do offers a useful insight. She suggests three main areas of mentor work: *supporting*, *challenging* and *providing vision*. Challenge and support are seen as mutually dependent and their relationship is illustrated in Figure 4.1. What is important for the mentor to know and recognise is that: 'What is support for one person may be challenge for another.' (Daloz 1986, p. 213). I suspect that it is only when there is a closeness between mentor and student that the mentor will be able to sense which is which and the student will feel able to attempt to articulate this. Indeed Brookfield (1987) talks of how important creating an atmosphere of trust is before one can start critically to question. With this need in mind I want to give attention to the particular elements raised by Daloz (1986). As they are often context specific what I intend to offer are practical examples of instances which were supportive, challenging or which provided vision.

Supporting

One of the strategies I have found helpful for some students is offering them feedback along the lines of *perceived strengths* and *areas to work*

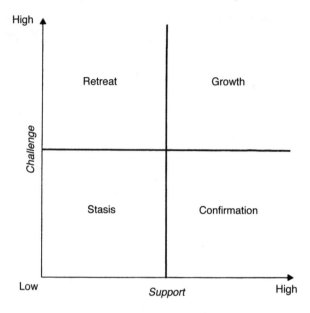

Fig. 4.1 The mutually dependent relationships in mentoring (after Daloz, L.A. (1986) *Effective Teaching and Mentoring: Realising the Transformation Power of Adult Learning Experiences*, (figure on p. 214), Jossey-Bass, London).

on (rather than 'strengths versus weaknesses'). This is in addition to their self assessment and reflects the feeling that positive feedback should come first (Northedge 1990) and will promote the student's self concept. It has been my experience that students really value constructive feedback which offers them insight into why something is or is not effective (Reid 1997). There is an issue of developing their own ability to do so but it is also related to experiencing it from others.

In one such feedback session with a student, Jan, I cautiously suggested that from observation I felt that she was unsure about using the ward telephone. This appeared to enable her to discuss how she felt afraid and consequently avoided being involved with its use, particularly when speaking to relatives. Given her response and her indication that it was an area she wanted to address we took it further.

After establishing how she felt we explored what might have contributed to these feelings. Jan identified an experience as a relative where she had been offered scant information. This led her to want to offer more than the bare minimum yet she recognised that she might not know the patient or relatives well enough, or not feel in a position to take that responsibility. From this I gently probed to elicit what was strong and what was weak about such a position. From this she could see that while it was a skill she did not yet have, her awareness of this deficit was vital as it prevented her from operating dangerously! From my feedback I was able to affirm how effective I generally found her communication skills with clients to be and why. We then explored the similarities and differences of communicating on the phone and doing so directly with clients.

From this we formed a plan of action which involved:

(1) Joint reflection on how I handled particular phone calls.
(2) Answering all incoming calls to the ward when she was available and directing them to the person concerned.
(3) Jan to note her level of discomfort when admitting that she did not know something but would find someone who did.

This plan was then reviewed at a later date and revised according to Jan's feeling of progress and need. What I was offering were probes to the process of reflection. I find constantly referring to the reflective cycle of Figure 4.2 from Gibbs (1988) very helpful with some students. That I was successful in this instance was in part due to the sense of awareness I had of who and where Jan was. For instance, some students may need to concentrate on unpicking what is actually happening in a situation.

As both Schön (1985) and Powell (1989) recognised, awareness of the experience and an ability to describe it are difficult though essential

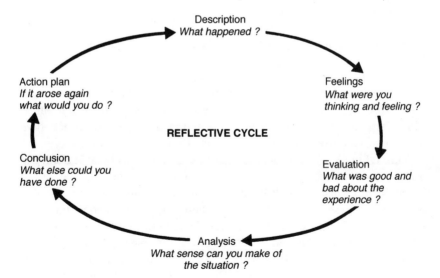

Fig. 4.2 The reflective cycle (from Gibbs 1988)

skills. The joint exploration of the cycle enables students to identify where they are in terms of their reflection, and reduces the risk of assumption or misdiagnosis on the part of the mentor. This is another way to increase your awareness as a mentor – you can ascertain what and how you know; or find an alternative route if you are wrong.

Although the process of identifying and addressing need within the reflective cycle can be slow, to leap stages may inhibit learning (Brookfield 1987) or ill equip mentees to transfer the process to other situations. I have experienced the temptation, either on mine or the mentee's part, to go for a 'quick fix' rather than see the development of reflection in the context of ongoing need. Given this proviso I feel that the exemplar demonstrates some of what Daloz (1986) outlines as being skills of supporting:

- listening
- providing structure
- expressing positive expectations
- serving as an advocate
- sharing ourselves
- making it special.

Such skills also apply not only to the development of reflection but also its management. As the students use reflection to evidence their learning the issue of how to handle it is important. Often the students find themselves in difficulties as they polarise around one of two extreme positions:

torrent of examples ⟵————⟶ cannot find an example

Often it is a question of learning to 'cash in' on experiences. While this may sound mercenary, it also promotes a richness of reflection in which one experience can be unpacked to expose so much. This has implications for promoting transferable skills and enabling the focus of reflection to move beyond the self (Goodman 1984).

Throughout such relationships the mentor needs to bear in mind the risk of over-identification with the student or being carried away in the excitement of discovery. It is all too easy to presume that just because you can analyse what is happening and see the potential, then the mentee will. To take over could create dependency but is more likely to inhibit learning for the student. There is also the risk that it will blind the mentor to the student's insights, which can be equally valid. Awareness of this as a potential risk is vital. One way to avoid this is to suspend belief or notions of a fixed outcome (the outcome can later be matched to the required outcome of competencies and aims). This offers a genuineness in the probing questions such as 'What is happening here?' and 'Where does that take you?' that feels helpful. In this way the process of reflection is the mentee's, yet the mentor can share in promoting it.

From the exemplar and the cautions that follow it becomes clear that support is not offered in isolation. For instance if I had not risked gently challenging Jan about the use of the telephone the opportunity for support and guidance in addressing it might have been lost, and so within the atmosphere of support challenge is considered.

Challenging

An instance where challenge was needed was in a relationship involving another student, Ruth. Initially Ruth appeared very quiet and almost timid and much of what I offered was in terms of support. One of Ruth's aims was to develop the skills of cleaning and dressing a wound. I was concerned at her concentration on the task, as it did not reflect the holistic nature of the intended learning, though in remembering myself as a student nurse I could understand it. After she had watched me dressing a client's wound several times, and had got to know the client, Mary, I suggested that Ruth ask Mary if she could perform the dressing. This she did, Mary agreed, and with me as a supportive onlooker, Ruth performed the dressing on her own and to Mary's satisfaction.

Following this Ruth expressed her sense of achievement at the successful completion of the task. While I reinforced this I felt that now was the time to take this further. I asked Ruth why the dressing had been successful. She found this difficult to answer except in technical terms. I posed two scenarios in which (1) she was to perform the dressing on a patient she did not know and (2) she was a patient who received fragmented care from different nurses, including a nurse she did not know, in the task of dressing her wound. Through this exploration Ruth was able to identify that it had been her relationship with Mary which had been the most significant factor in the successful dressing performance.

A second example is one that occurred with Jan. As the shift progressed it was obvious that Jan had a considerable workload and was tired. Mid-shift she mentioned how she had been distracted from her work the night before and needed to do more before a session on the computer the following day. She then suggested missing the next day's early shift that we had negotiated she would work. Internally my reactions were:

- sympathy to her plight. Jan was generally well organised and ahead with her work (knowing her helped)

- knowing that it was not an easy thing for her to suggest and I did not want to appear inflexible
- feeling strongly that although she was supernumerary at present, when she qualified she would need to have a work ethos to fulfill her commitment.

My response to Jan was to say 'OK, if that really has to be' but I then asked what she would do if she was working in employment. Jan admitted that she could not have that choice then. In recognising this awareness I offered a flexible response of going early that night in order to be able to come in the next morning. As it was she stayed working in the coffee room from 7 p.m. until I left and achieved what she wanted to do while still remaining near the clinical environment. Jan's own comment on the situation was: 'A compromise was achieved and through Brigid I was made aware of my supernumerary status and its potential for misuse.'

In examining these examplars there are direct issues of challenging involved. In his work on promoting critical thinking Brookfield (1987) defines it as:

(1)   identifying and challenging assumptions
(2)   imagining and exploring alternatives.

Daloz (1986) writes of ways of enabling the students to grow through working to close the distance in the relationship that the mentor deliberately creates. She discusses:

- setting tasks
- heating up dichotomies
- setting high standards
- constructive hypotheses
- engaging in discussions.

Indeed these skills are involved in what I have recounted. However there are also more factors involved:

(1)   *The timing of the challenge.* This involves not just the immediate context; that is, is it a good or a bad time, but also that within the relationship. Brookfield (1987) talks of earning the right to challenge that involves trust building as explored earlier.
(2)   *A sense of congruency.* What is being asked of the mentee is nothing that the mentor would not ask of themselves. For example for the mentor to be known as a nurse who asks the mentee, 'What if?', and articulates his or her own standards and goals.

(3) *The skill of risk taking.* From personal reflection this involves the consistency of the relationship and how it has developed, the recognition of opportunities, knowing the student's aims and trusting your own judgement.

(4) *The way it is done.* Again I return to the issue of support. One of the concepts mentors often find most challenging is that of challenging students! I feel it is closely related to the skills of giving positive feedback. The issues are related because both involve specificity about either what is effective (Gray & Gerrard 1977) or the challenge being set. Further, both flourish if the two key elements of support and challenge are present. Again the fine balance and interrelationship between the two elements, as seen in Daloz's diagram (Fig. 4.1), are invoked.

Providing vision

Daloz (1986, p. 230) describes vision as:

> 'The context that hosts both support and challenge in the service of transformation.'

Providing vision involves issues of reflective attitudes (Goodman 1984) and the belief in the juxtaposition of the other two key elements of the mentor's role, those of challenge and support. Most importantly vision is a metaphor for greater understanding. While this may involve using role models it needs to move beyond this. The mentor is only effective if the object of inspiration is nursing, not just the mentor. This is where the model in which a student has multiple sequential (note not concurrent) mentors throughout her or his course can have advantages. In the same way that each client is unique so is each nurse and her or his vision of nursing.

There is also an analogy of 'offering a map' (Daloz 1986), which is similar to the concept of being a 'skilled companion' as Campbell (1984) names the nurse in her/his role with clients. The issue is that of enabling a journey. The mentor/nurse has a clear idea of the terrain yet it is the mentee/client who should be the determinant of the destination. The skill involved is in knowing the type of companionship to offer in each role. That will depend on the mentee or the client. The mentor can not necessarily avoid the pitfalls inherent in such journeys. Rather the mentor can enable the mentee to: 'know better when she is in one – and thus take fuller advantage of the unique opportunities that most pitfalls offer' (Daloz 1986, p. 208).

While exploring my own and other's experiences of being a mentor and drawing from them the key elements of the role, it is interesting to consider how that role is defined and perceived by others.

Being a mentor

'In practical terms the mentor was perceived to make or break the placement for students by determining how much students got to do and learn and how welcome they felt'.

(Reid 1997, p. 141)

The term mentor is one that has received considerable attention in the last decade within nursing education. Numerous articles debate what the term actually means, for example Coates & Gormley (1997), Maggs (1994). These range from a long-term chosen professional who acts as a guide for a lesser experienced professional, that is career mentor, to an allocated qualified nurse who oversees a student's specific clinical experience for a short period of time. As identified by many researchers there is little consensus of opinion about the components of mentors' roles and few significant studies (Atkins & Williams 1995). Even the English National Board (ENB) appears to have difficulty in maintaining a consistent definition (cited by Cahil 1996) initially as:

'A person selected by the student to assist, advise and counsel (but who will not normally be involved in the formal supervision or assessment of that particular student)'

(ENB 1988)

then as

'an appropriately qualified and experienced first level nurse/midwife/health visitor who, by example and facilitation guides, assists and supports the practitioner in learning new skills, adopting new behaviours and acquiring new attitudes.'

(ENB 1990)

This disparity of concept usage may relate to what Philips *et al.* (1996), in their study of pre-registration nurse education in Wales, called 'a resilient attachment to the word mentor in clinical areas throughout Wales' (p. 1082), in the face of the official use of the term 'preceptor' which is defined by the Welsh National Board for Nursing, Midwifery and Health Visiting (WNB) as follows:

'For situations in which a student in a practice area is assigned to a staff nurse for the duration of the allocation, in which the two work parallel shifts, and in which the student is supported as he or she works towards the planned learning outcomes for the placement, we would suggest the term preceptor.'

(WNB 1992)

Woodrow (1994) in an otherwise confusing paper suggests that

'playing semantics without addressing the practical problems of implementation leaves already stretched practitioners often holding no qualifications in education to interpret confusion.'

(Woodrow 1994, p. 817)

Therefore, although mindful of Maggs' (1994) concern that uncritical adoption of a term that has several meanings can lead to a dilution of principles or their inappropriate use, it is important to offer a clear definition of the term mentor in this chapter. The work of Atkins & Williams (1995) and Spouse (1996) offers defining features of the mentor as used within practice areas associated with the Oxford Brookes University undergraduate nursing programme. The mentor is defined as a qualified nurse who has, in negotiation with a lecturer practitioner (LP) or link lecturer, agreed to have a student assigned to her or him for the duration of a clinical module. The mentor is responsible for facilitating opportunities for the students to achieve their learning objectives and relevant competencies and for validating the achievement of the latter.

The mentor is responsible for guiding the students' learning in the clinical area by:

- Initially being with the student on days of the clinical placement and liaising with co-mentors if necessary.
- Contracting and encouraging the student to self assess and identify objectives to be met during the placement ensuring that such objectives are relevant to their previous experiences and relevant to the competencies that are to be achieved in the module.
- Discussing and agreeing the resources and strategies required for their learning including how they will access the LP/lecturer linked to the practice area.
- Planning the learning experiences so that the modular competencies can be achieved.
- Encouraging self assessment by the student and assessing the learning outcomes yourself, ensuring there is adequate evidence to support both the student's assessment and yours of his or her achievement.
- Identifying and ensuring opportunities are made for students to

reflect on their experiences; initially this is envisaged happening at the end of each shift.

- Encouraging the students' recording of their experiences as soon as possible after the event by recording in their personal log/diary.
- Using their lecturer practitioner/lecturer and the student's personal tutor for advice or information as necessary.

From this it can be seen that the role is one which Donovan (1990) refers to as 'restricted mentoring'. In this the emphasis is on a short-term interaction (four to thirteen weeks) concentrating on the educational needs of the student; in this case clinical competence, development and validation. The mentor is a first level clinical nurse (ENB 1988) and the relationship is focused and intense (Fields 1991) due to the nature of working together. Bracken & Davis (1989) raise the potential difficulty of the mentors having to make themselves available. However in my experience students, in accordance with the course philosophy, are expected to fit in with their mentors off duty. With the exception of extensive night duty or holidays this is not unrealistic and it is in the student's interest to ensure that this is achieved.

From the available literature there is no doubt that the role of mentor is viewed as a significant one in the students' clinical learning (e.g. Philips *et al.* 1996). This key role is the case even if it is related to negative experiences (Cahil 1996), which only serve to demonstrate the power of mentors; one student defined being dependent 'on mentors' good opinion' (Baines 1995). This key role is also apparent in the plethora of studies regarding the role of the nurse teacher in clinical practice, for example Carlisle *et al.* (1997). As Forrest *et al.* (1996) identified:

'Students ... were of the unanimous opinion that the most effective teachers of clinical nursing skills were the trained nurses working in the clinical areas'

(Forrest *et al.* 1996, p. 1261)

From studies available, the qualities of a mentor that mentors and students appeared to value were those of teaching and supporting, with the use of terms like befriending (Spouse 1996, Anforth 1992), supporting (Atkins & Williams 1995) and coaching (Spouse 1996).

However it appears that opinion is divided as to whether the role of the mentor should encompass that of assessing students. With regard to this, Anforth (1992) reported the ENB stance that mentors are 'not normally assessors', though Clifford (1994) and While (1991) identified that they often are. While (1991) tempered this observation about mentors with the caution that 'their skills in clinical evaluation have not been subject to a rigorous analysis' (p. 452) and an American study identified that 'preceptors' perceived their primary responsibility was to teach rather than evaluate (Ferguson 1996). Indeed their finding was that

> 'they indicated their discomfort with the process of evaluating student behaviour for a grade or a promotion though comfortable with informal evaluation or feedback.'

> (Ferguson 1996, p. 59)

Many authors are of the opinion that the role of assessing students is not compatible with mentoring, for example Woodrow (1994) and this has been identified in several studies (Coates & Gormley 1997), Duke 1996). However, when the role of mentor as assessor is questioned no alternative person is proposed and it appears in practice that most mentors in the UK are assessors (Woodrow 1995, Clifford 1994).

The reasons cited for questioning mentors undertaking the role of assessors were as follows:

- it conflicted with their already heavy workload (Coates & Gormley 1997, Rogers & Lawton 1995)
- their lack of educational preparation (Davies *et al.* 1996, Forrest *et al.* 1996, Philips *et al.* 1996, Rogers & Lawton 1995)
- the perceived conflict with the supportive aspects of the role (Duke 1996, Oldmeadow 1996, Atkins & Williams 1995)

In an Australian account of how student physiotherapists' competency is assessed Oldmeadow (1996) questioned whether the qualified practitioners were doubtful, and therefore anxious, about their abilities fearing that they could be either under-rating students or allowing those who shouldn't to 'slip through'. In Duke's (1996) study of Australian clinical teachers and their role in clinical evaluation, she notes that they reported 'gut feelings' about students but that it 'seems from their responses that they did not feel that it was legitimate to act upon them when considering student performance' (Duke 1996, p. 411). Duke attributed this reluctance of teachers to trust their judgement as a symptom of 'oppressed behaviour' and inadequate preparation for the role.

The apparent reluctance on the part of some mentors to 'fail' or give negative feedback to students was identified by Lankshear (1990) who felt it to be related to a difficulty in pinpointing their judgement in skills other than psychomotor ones (Duke 1996 also). In addition Lankshear (1990) noted a concern for the consequences in terms of confidence for the students that any 'fail' or feedback of concern would have. This concern for students was identified as a conflict with the caregiver role of the nurse (Paterson & Crawford 1994, based on a cited study by Paterson (1991)), where clinical teachers exhibited signs of grief when required to fail a student. However, such a contention needs to be considered with respect to the current expectations of qualified nurses which involve monitoring and evaluating themselves and colleagues in order to promote quality. It would be interesting to imagine the response ward managers might provoke if they felt that they could not be involved in their staff's performance reviews on account of their supportive role with staff (or vice versa). If the reaction to challenging situations is one of abdication, then the profession's ability to deal with the 'swampy low lands' of practice would be in question.

In their recent ENB funded study Hallet *et al.* (1996) found assessment, for students and their mentors, to be a key stage in what they identified as the learning career of the students within a placement. From their findings it appeared an activity for which the mentors felt equipped; though the formal educational assessment they were required to complete, in addition to their own monitoring of the students, was felt to frequently fail to 'reflect the reality of the students' experience'. From Hallet *et al.*'s study two issues arise: (1) if an assessment is perceived as unrealistic how relevant and therefore valid will it be for students and mentors? (2) the mentor participants were district nurses and it would be interesting to know why their educational background appears to have equipped them better than participants in other reported studies. It may well be that they have had additional education to be clinical practice teachers (CPTs) in order to facilitate the learning of district nursing students. Not only is the preparation to be a CPT of significant duration, it is essential for the mentor role of post-registration nurses studying to become district nurses. In 'reward' for this role CPTs often receive a higher pay grade and are supposed to have reduced clinical caseloads.

The student participants in my study (Reid 1997) placed an emphasis on 'getting competencies' and as a result they appeared to focus on 'doing' activities in order to 'get' competencies. However it was apparent that 'doing' in itself did not count for the students unless they could articulate what they had done and have this validated by their mentor. Thus being able to express themselves through writing and their actions being visible to their mentors appeared to them as the main requirements of the system. Students appeared to feel that their ability to write was not necessarily commensurate with their ability in practice and that their mentors were not always available, either because of other work demands or because of their adopted mode of working with students. This feeling led the students to view the system as unfair.

In the mentor role defined in this chapter there is an active element implied in the activities outlined. Although there is a natural concern for the outcome (e.g. validation of competencies and written assessment reflecting a practice marked by lecturer practitioner/lecturer) much of the role should focus on the process; developing and managing reflection. It is only by exploring what it means to be a reflective mentor, and some of the strategies available, that insight as to *how* the activities on the list of mentor responsibilities can be gained.

From the experiences I have outlined in the chapter, the relationship I have described is often a close one. Indeed in rejecting Burnard's (1990) suggestion that a more detached relationship would serve the purpose better, I feel that it is the development of trust and getting to know each other that can provide an effective foundation.

Forming the relationship

There have been criticisms of the mentor/mentee relationship with regard to the short time span afforded to it (Donovan 1990, Barlow 1991) and the lack of choice in the relationship (Bracken & Davis 1989). In counteracting such criticisms I find the parallel of the development of a trusting and effective nurse/patient relationship strong. Such a relationship may occur within the space of hours and rarely has a degree of choice in it. The key factors of this relationship building are ones of intent, commitment and atmosphere of purpose (Meutzel 1988). Although recognising that the mentor/mentee relationship is different to the nurse/patient one in scope and aim, it is useful for the mentor to build on the skills she or he already possesses as a relationship builder.

Schön (1985) writes of needing a setting of low risk for the student to practise in. While this could be interpreted as a purely physical environment (such as the clinical room in a School of Nursing), within the real world of practice in which students find themselves it is offered in supernumerary status and the relationship of the students with their mentors. Both Daloz (1986) and Brookfield (1987) refer to the creation of trust as a necessary starting point.

Upon meeting the mentee I try to create an atmosphere of trust and establish mutual expectations. How this occurs is very dependent on the individual mentee and how I'm feeling and as ever, the degree of my self awareness is important. For example I may have to tone down my zeal or compensate for fatigue, these being two regular attributes of my mode of work! I invite them to tell me how they have previously worked (clinically and with regard to their learning contracts) and to articulate, if they can, their preferred learning style. It is by this means that I attempt to establish what is supportive or challenging for them. For example, one student preferred negotiated and reviewed short-term goals, whereas another felt that this was intrusive and wanted to go it alone for longer. A mentor cannot promise to be all things to all mentees, however they can be aware of needs and adopt their style in a way that feels congruent to them.

While establishing the mentees' needs it is important that an element of reciprocity occurs. I outline what I have to offer to the mentees; my needs and my expectations of them. This may involve personal disclosure on my part and indication of my perceived weaknesses such as a tendency to expect too much too soon. There is a danger that disclosure may inhibit the mentee or reduce confidence in the mentor. However the projection of credibility and willingness to share have generally felt effective to me.

Whilst the aim of the relationship is to support and manage reflection there has to be an element of congruence throughout the relationship. Reflection is not something one should switch on as a discrete entity. In his study on working towards a theory of reflection, Goodman (1984) turned to the work of Dewey and Van Manen to offer three mutually dependent elements:

- the focus of reflection
- the process of reflection
- attitudes to reflection

In clarifying what constitutes reflective attitudes, Goodman (1984) discusses:

(1) *open mindedness* in which things are not taken for granted, and self questioning is promoted
(2) *responsibility* to make sense of diverse ideas and to move beyond questions of immediate utility
(3) *wholeheartedness* in which self esteem and commitment are seen as important and enabling in risk taking.

With this view of reflective attitudes and the need for congruency, I find it helps to extend the relationship formation to the clarification of practical roles. This is particularly important when the mentee is a student who is supernumerary. Mentees need to clarify the commitment they expect, for example to me, our patients and, the nursing team. In exploring their role with respect to me, I have found that most students move along a continuum, the pace varying according to their experience and developmental rate. This continuum of the developing roles of the mentees can be shown as:

Shadows
needing to feel comfortable and competent with
being with clients
being in the area
watching/shadowing the mentor

Extensions of the mentor
needing to feel comfortable and competent with
giving care under direct supervision
they may need prompting

↓

Partners with the mentor
needing to feel comfortable and competent with
caring for a client with minimal supervision
they may need parameters to work within

The articulation of expectations does not guarantee a smooth journey, but usually promotes an atmosphere in which problems on either side can be addressed. There also needs to be recognition of a realistic pacing of the journey. As Vaughan & FitzGerald (1992) observed with regard to reflection: 'Indeed to try to achieve such a level of enquiry all the time in everyday practice would be utterly exhausting and cumbersome and in itself might constrain creativity.' (p. 145)

In the study I undertook (Reid 1997) the lecturer practitioner participants identified the mentors as having the key role in the assessment of competence. The role of the mentor involved what was perceived as the 'sanctioning' of the student's performance. This process of sanctioning was apparent in the following ways:

- Formal validation of students 'competence' was required, as described by one lecturer/practitioner as 'written evidence which is validated by the mentor of the competencies that the student needs to acquire'.
- Informal endorsement throughout the students time in clinical practice. For example a student participant spoke of mentors saying 'yes ... I'm happy that you are competent to do this'. This aspect was also observable in the actions of mentors when they 'allowed' students to do things.
- As an ally whereby mentors were perceived as 'backing up' or confirming what students had written that they had achieved.

Mentors themselves appeared aware of their responsibility in this role of assessment to ensure safe practice. Their reference to 'checking up' or not signing competencies if they were concerned implied that they took this responsibility seriously. One mentor, Jan, articulated this when she said 'it's a big responsibility' and explained that she wanted to be fairly balanced, because 'I don't want to upset her by being too hard and on the other hand if I've been too soft, I don't want her to think she's wonderful when she's not'. However this mentor did wonder if her opinion was relied on too much.

From all participants, though, there were expressions of doubt as to what was expected in the role of the mentor:

- Mentors themselves spoke of uncertainty about aspects of their role. This was apparent when a mentor referred to whether he should have fedback his thoughts on her apparent 'over confidence' to a student saying, 'I'm not sure that's my role to do that'.
- As student participants identified, the general view about mentors was to question whether some mentors knew what they were doing.
- Even lecturer practitioners had doubts as one voiced when she said 'I sometimes worry that mentors will validate student's competencies because they are unsure of what else to do'. This was echoed by another's view that mentors need permission to be able to say when they feel someone isn't competent.

In terms of the mentors' experience and preparation there appeared to be considerable variation. A student participant wondered how people assessed competence. She felt that: '... as you get through your training you pick more up ... but whether it's just by luck or by judgement is a hard thing to judge'.

It was apparent that mentors' previous learning experiences informed how they themselves wanted to be. One mentor spoke of how she remembered mentors who had not had time for her. She said that they had either 'been too busy to explain things or been too stressed'. Another mentor spoke of how his various experiences as a student had informed him. He said:

'I had some good mentors when I was a student one or two lousy ones as well. I remember how awful it was ... feeling frustrated and couldn't really ... assert yourself ... 'I want this' you know. You can't afford to fall out with your mentor or anyone else on the ward really ... So I remember how bad that was and how good it was ... to go on to another ward where teachers who were mentors were very good you know I vowed not to get my students into that sort of situation.'

The third mentor participant recounted what amounted to an apprenticeship:

'I did the traditional nurse training, qualified and came here 4 years ago. And it was the old fashioned sort where you were first year students with a third year student. Right? And facilitator. So you learnt. I had both experiences, they still influence me ... I can remember my facilitator doing some teaching with me and talking through what had happened and what was going on and how I felt I was doing. You take all those positive things and use them. And then of course when I became a third year student I had first year students to teach ... Having somebody work alongside me. And teaching them as I go so that the ongoing teaching part, the difference between being a teacher and a mentor, the teaching part is quite easy but the mentoring ... [was more difficult].'

From the available research of students' and mentors' experiences it is obvious that if mentors are to make a positive difference to the process of reflection and learning their needs must be actively considered.

The mentor's needs

The role of mentor articulated in this chapter is skilled and involves commitment and energy on the part of the practitioner. It is therefore appropriate to consider how the mentor develops and sustains her or his self. There are several categories of need: *preparation, support* and *reward*.

Preparation

Nurse registration education has until now offered little formal experience in the skills of facilitating learning. That is not to say that practitioners will not have developed them, but to note that it cannot be assumed. The practitioner who is to become a mentor needs to have several requisites:

- to want to become a mentor
- to be comfortable and competent in his or her present role
- to feel open to learning
- to have an awareness of the richness of practice and to value it.

Some have suggested formal qualifications as a basis for becoming a mentor, for example the ENB 998, (Morle 1990, Bracken & Davis 1989). The acceptability of such courses depends on the focus and depth of their scope and thus needs exploring. These may have a role but it is perhaps an ability to learn rather than to teach that has the greater influence (Schön 1985). Personally it has been the development of my own *reflective skills* initially within the support of a Certificate in Further

Education and used within clinical supervision that has been particularly useful.

All the mentors participating in the study I undertook (Reid 1997) had trained in different areas to the site of the study. From the perspective of the students there was an issue that there needed to be more preparation for mentors. The student participant said that:

> 'I think there needs to be more training for the lecturer practitioners and the mentors ... I mean, we've often talked about when we qualify what we will do as mentors and I said, but we know what not to do. You know I think the ones that have come through this system will make reasonably good mentors because they've seen the good and the bad side of it. Whereas a lot of the mentors are traditionally trained nurses. I mean what really made me laugh is that I was at [another placement] I said to [her mentor] are you in today, no I've got to go on my one, ONE day mentors course. And I'd been there 3 weeks!'

The mentor participants themselves admitted that they had not undergone any formal preparation for the role. One mentor had been qualified for two and a half years. In this time he had mentored several times though he had not had any formal preparation. This mentor talked of a module he would be doing the following term and said 'hopefully that will improve my skills'. Another mentor found it difficult to identify what had prepared her. She said:

> 'It's a bit unprepared ... I don't know what's prepared me as a mentor. I haven't had students before ... but I was an associate nurse and my last job had students, so I've always worked with them on the ward so I suppose ... I was aware of the students there'

The third mentor participant recalled that her preparation had occurred as she undertook to mentor her first student and how it had consisted of a one to one discussion with her lecturer practitioner about what was expected of her, the stage the students would be at and the system they were in.

With regard to educational preparation of mentors, Davies *et al.* (1996), in an ENB funded study, identified that any preparation consisted of either the ENB 998 course 'Teaching and assessing' or an in house course usually of two days duration focusing on the interpretation and completion of relevant assessment documentation. In a positional paper Harding & Greig (1994) made the assertion that mentors have 'been invested with an authority of which they are unaware and for which they are unprepared' (p. 118). Davies *et al.*'s (1996) findings identified that an area in which practitioners felt particularly unprepared was the assessment of practice as exemplified by the following: 'I am not quite sure how it (assessment of student practice) works. I've yet to have that explained to me. But my student assures me he knows how it is done' (Mentor, Mental Health Branch, Davies *et al.* 1996, p. 24).

Certainly some formal preparation specific to the role of mentor, both at the outset and then as a development tool is essential. This needs to address two factors, the interpersonal skills role and the organisational role. The former should consider reflection and the strategies I have outlined. The latter needs to encompass the mentees' course, their goals and what is expected of them. My initial preparation involved a session in which I reflected on people who had been significant in my development and the skills they had. Another useful approach is to examine varying learning styles within a group to gain an awareness of how individuals differ. In my preparation an invitation for us to construct our own learning contracts to use to focus our early reflections generated the following personal objectives:

(1)   to balance my roles as a patient caregiver, senior nurse on a shift and mentor
(2)   to feel a competence and ease in challenging students when necessary.

My needs of preparation continued to be met through close contact with the lecturer practitioner who was responsible for my mentor preparation and the students' clinical placements. With the lecturer practitioner I was able to have a supervisory relationship (as discussed in Bev Gillings' chapter, Chapter 5) in which I could reflect on my experience as a mentor in order to develop my skills. The integrated nature of the role of lecturer practitioner, who has close contact with both parties in the clinical setting, therefore could promote the development of mentors by ensuring that their needs are given continued attention.

Support for the mentor

Support can be offered formally through those involved in the course, either the lecturer practitioners/lecturers or mentor support groups. Being in supervision as a practitioner offers further aid particularly in learning to become self reflective. Often the question 'how do you know when you've been effective?' is asked of practitioners, and mentors should not be exempt. Through reflection and reception of the appropriate balance of support and challenge I can attempt to ascertain my effectiveness. It can sometimes be enticing to rely on feelings of being liked as testimony to effect. As Brookfield (1987) highlights in cautioning against this, some learning involves frustration and so possible discomfort. Finding mechanisms to discern these factors and to accommodate them while retaining self esteem can be facilitated through supervision.

In terms of nurses' workload, many studies have observed that it is increasing and that the role of mentor both adds to this and conflicts with it (e.g. Wilson-Barnett *et al.* 1995). There are, however, significant observations that need to temper this issue of mentor work overload. Spouse (1996) noted that some mentors were able to juggle their time well, which may be related to Atkins & Williams (1995) finding that mentors' ability to do this related to how integral they perceived mentoring to be to their role and how much control they had over their workload. Atkins & Williams identified that 'those participants with a real commitment to mentoring appearing less concerned about their mentoring role competing for their time with other nursing activities' (Atkins & Williams 1995, p. 1010). This links with the findings of Philips *et al.* (1996), that a key attribute to mentoring is motivation enabling the mentors in their study to be perceived as supportive even when they were stretched – which they frequently were.

Associated to mentors' ability to manage the role are the findings of Wilson-Barnett *et al.* (1995) who identified the support of colleagues and the approach to the organisation of nursing care to be factors which enhanced their learning and enjoyment of placements. This need for mentor support was also identified in a Canadian study of nurse preceptors (Dibert & Goldenberg 1995). The available studies would suggest that this support needs to be both organisational (to manage the role) and educational (to develop the role beyond the current 'starters' boost).

The organisations, both of practice and education, need to recognise and value the role of mentor. Although they are not able to reward it materially, values can be transmitted through behaviour and affect self esteem and so the commitment of those involved. Support from colleagues as they recognise the increased demands on the mentor is invaluable. This does not necessarily involve taking over aspects of the mentor's practice; simply demonstrating an awareness that support could be needed and promoting teamwork is usually sufficient. Another source of support is often the clients, both to the mentees and mentor; I have often been boosted by their interest, tolerance and an attitude, that such a role is somehow special.

Reward

I think it is important to ask 'what do I get out of this?' The potential of motivation is one of the vital elements ensuring the success of the role.

As registered nurses, the development of other nurses is inherent to our role but never before has this been so instrumental and demanding. From personal and anecdotal evidence, supported by Tongue (1992) there is a strong element of reciprocity in the relationship. Tongue's respondents commented on what they had learnt from their students. This learning encompasses not only new knowledge transmitted from students but increased insight into and an ability to be reflective about what we do as practitioners.

The findings of my study (Reid 1997) described the role of mentor as one that the staff nurses expected to take on as part of their responsibilities. In this respect the role is as described by Atkins & Williams (1995) when they undertook a study within the same pre-registration nurse education programme. The concept of a mentor as a qualified nurse, to whom individual students are allocated to for the duration of a clinical module, that Atkins & Williams (1995) described, does not appear dissimilar to other roles of mentor/preceptor described within the UK. It was apparent in my study that normally the student negotiates to work the same shifts as their mentor to undertake the minimum number of clinical hours required in the module. It was also important to note that in the module handbook, great emphasis was placed on the students' responsibilities to seek out and use learning opportunities and to respect the time constraints their mentors may face.

I also found that the ways in which the students experienced 'working with' their mentors varied (Reid 1997). The quality and quantity of 'working with' mentors and students appeared to be affected by their availability to each other and their implicit style of working. Their styles of working together reflected the styles of collaboration between mentors and students identified by Spouse (1996) within the same programme of pre-registration nurse education. Such evidence indicates that preparation and support of mentors is likely to enhance factors such as reciprocity of learning and hence rewards for the role.

It would appear that the role of the community practice teacher (CPT), as mentor to post-registration nurses studying to become district nurses, is one which holds less ambiguity and requires specific recognised preparation (Goding 1997) in comparison with the concerns outlined in the preceding paragraphs. As discussed earlier in this chapter the factors of recognition and reward associated with the CPT role may be significant in enabling it to continue and in the perception that it is effective. Further work regarding the CPT role and how it could inform generic mentor preparation could prove useful.

Feedback from students should be examined to aid learning about being a mentor. It is very tempting to dismiss the less positive or to gain a quick fix from glowing accolades without exploring either further. As practitioners we often miss so much by accepting things at face value, a classic example being our acceptance of 'nurse you are wonderful' without trying to find out why a particular patient feels this.

On commenting on how supportive she found a ward environment to be, a student I worked with responded to my question of 'I wonder what makes it so?' She did this by creating an objective in her learning contract about it. The evidence she provided was a very useful perspective to have for those of us so immersed in it. Additionally in the development of a frequently close relationship there is often a great deal of practical and emotional support from the students that should not be under-estimated. However the degree to which the students are felt to be supportive depends on their approach and the mentor's feeling of comfort in the examination of her or his practice.

Summary

The development of my skills through varied role experience, particularly as a clinical supervisor and researcher has enabled me to develop my original exploration of the role of mentor. Mentorship is about negotiating a journey of learning through action and reflection. This chapter has offered practical strategies to underpin the philosophy of what I believe is a powerful educational tool. I have highlighted that the instrumental factor in the role of mentor is self awareness and use of self. If consideration is given to the preparation and the needs of the role then practitioners can gain a chance to develop themselves and their understanding of nursing. If this is combined with an awareness of learners' individual needs, there is the potential for the ongoing balance of challenge and support to be facilitated in a journey of joint discovery. My journeys have not been without pitfalls, yet I believe the effect of each has been to enhance my understanding of myself and nursing in some way. The fulfilment of also enabling another in their development is a significant reward. The potential benefits of this mutual development indicate that such a role requires further consideration and opportunity in the growth of the professional practitioner.

References

Anforth, P. (1992) Mentors not assessors. *Nurse Education Today*, **12**, 299–302.
Atkins, S. & Williams, A. (1995) Registered nurses' experiences of mentoring undergraduate nursing students. *Journal of Advanced Nursing*, **21**, 1006–15.
Baines, E. (1995) Nor mentor be? *Nursing Standard*, **9** (21), 54.

Barlow, S. (1991) Impossible dream. *Nursing Times*, **87** 153-4

Berger, P. & Luckman, T. (1967) *The Social Construction of Reality*, Penguin, London.

Boyd E.M. & Fales, A.W. (1983) Reflective learning: key to learning from experience. *Journal of Humanistic Psychology*, **23** (2), 99–117.

Bracken, E. & Davis, J. (1989) The implication of mentorship in nursing career development. *Senior Nurse*, **9** (5), 15–16.

Brookfield, S.D. (1987) *Developing Critical Thinkers*, Open University Press, Milton Keynes.

Burnard, P. (1990) The student experience: adult learning and mentorship revisited. *Nurse Education Today*, **10**, 349–54.

Cahil H.A. (1996) A qualitative analysis of student nurses' experiences of mentorship. *Journal of Advanced Nursing*, **24**, 791–9.

Campbell, A. (1984) *Moderated Love: a Theology of Professional Care*, Society for the Propagation of Christian Knowledge, London.

Carlisle, C., Kirk, S. & Luker K. (1997) The clinical role of nurse teachers within a Project 2000 course framework. *Journal of Advanced Nursing*, **25**, 386–95.

Clifford, C. (1994) Assessment of clinical practice and the role of the nurse teacher. *Nurse Education Today*, **14**, 272–9.

Coates, V.E. & Gormley, E. (1997) Learning the practice of nursing: views about preceptorship. *Nurse Education Today*, **17**, 91–8.

Daloz, L.A. (1986) *Effective Teaching and Mentoring*, Jossey-Bass, London.

Davies, S., White, E., Riley, E. & Twinn, S. (1996) How can nurse teachers be more effective in practice settings? *Nurse Education Today*, **16**, 19–27.

Dibert, C. & Goldenberg, D. (1995) Preceptors' perceptions of benefits, rewards, supports and commitment to the preceptor role. *Journal of Advanced Nursing*, **21**, 1144–51.

Donovan, J. (1990) The concept and role of mentor. *Nurse Education Today*, **10**, 294–8.

Duke M. (1996) Clinical evaluation – difficulties experienced by sessional clinical teachers of nursing: a qualitative study. *Journal of Advanced Nursing*, **23**, 408–14.

ENB (1990) Regulations & Guidelines for the Approval of Institutions & Courses 1990, ENB, London.

ENB (1998) Circular 1998/39/APS Institutional and course approval/re-approval process, information required, *Criteria and Guidelines*, English National Board, London.

Ferguson, L.M. (1996) Preceptors enhance students' self confidence. *Nursing Connections*, **9** (1), 49–61.

Fields, W.L. (1991) Mentoring in nursing: a historical approach. *Nursing Outlook*, **39** (6), 257–61.

Forrest M., Brown N. & Pollock L. (1996) The clinical role of the nurse teacher: an exploratory study of the nurse teachers' present and ideal role in the clinical area. *Journal of Advanced Nursing*, **24**, 1257–64.

Gibbs, G. (1988) *Learning by Doing: A guide to teaching and learning methods*, Further Education Unit, Oxford Polytechnic (now Oxford Brookes University), Oxford.

Goding, L.A. (1997) Can degree level practice be assessed? *Nurse Education Today*, **17**, 158–61.

Goodman, J. (1984) Reflection and teacher education: A case study and theoretical analysis. *Interchange*, **15** (3), 9–26.

Gray, W.A. & Gerrard, B.A. (1977) *Learning by Doing: Developing Teaching Skills*, Addison-Wesley, London.

Hallet, C.E., Williams, A. & Butterworth, T. (1996) The learning career in the community setting: a phenomenological study of a Project 2000 placement. *Journal of Advanced Nursing*, **23**, 578–86.

Harding, C. & Greig, M. (1994) Issues of accountability in the assessment of practice. *Nurse Education Today*, **14**, 118–23.

Jarvis, P. (1992) Reflective practice and nursing. *Nurse Education Today*, **12**, 174–81.

Lankshear, A. (1990) Failure to fail: the teacher's dilemma. *Nursing Standard*, **4** (20), 35–7.

Maggs, C. (1994) Mentorship in nursing and midwifery education: issues for research. *Nurse Education Today*, **14**, 22–9.

Meutzel, P.A. (1988) Therapeutic nursing. In Pearson, A. (ed) (1988) *Primary Nursing*, Croom Helm, London.

Morle, K.M.F. (1990) Mentorship – is it a case of the emperor's new clothes, or just a rose by any other name? *Nurse Education Today*, **10**, 66-9.

Northedge, N. (1990) *The Good Study Guide*, Open University Press, Milton Keynes.

Oldmeadow, L. (1996) Developing clinical competence: a mastery pathway. *Australian Physiotherapy*, **42** (1), 37–44.

Paterson, B. & Crawford, M. (1994) Caring in nursing education: an analysis. *Journal of Advanced Nursing*, **19**, 164–73.

Philips, R.M., Davies, N.B. & Neary, M. (1996) The practitioner-teacher: a study in the introduction of mentors in the pre registration nurse education programme in Wales part 2.' *Journal of Advanced Nursing*, **23**, 1080–88.

Philips, T., Schostak, J., Bedford, H. & Robinson, J. (1993) Assessment of Competencies in Nursing & Midwifery Education and Training (the Ace project). *ENB Research Highlights*, October 1993.

Powell, J.H. (1989) The reflective practitioner in nursing. *Journal of Advanced Nursing*, **14**, 824–32.

Reid B. (1997) An exploration of the assessment of competence in undergraduate nursing students. Unpublished M.Phil, University of Reading.

Rogers, P. & Lawton, C. (1995) Self assessment of Project 2000 supervision. *Nursing Times*, **91** (27), 42–5.

Schön, D. (1985) *Educating the Reflective Practitioner*, Jossey-Bass, San Francisco.

Spouse, J. (1996) The effective mentor: a model for student centred learning. *Nursing Times*, **92** (13), 32–5.

Tongue, C. (1992) Mentorship: what is it and does it work? Unpublished paper given at the Institute of Nursing, Oxford, 22nd October 1992.

Vaughan, B. & Fitzgerald, M. (1992) *Knowledge for Nursing Practice*, Butterworth Heinemann, Oxford.

While, A. (1991) The problem of clinical evaluation – a review. *Nurse Education Today*, **11**, 448–53.

Wilson-Barnett, J., Butterworth, T., White, E., Twinn, S., Davies, S. & Riley, E. (1995) Clinical support and the Project 2000 nursing student: factors influencing this process. *Journal of Advanced Nursing*, **21**, 1152–8.

WNB (1992) Mentors, Preceptors & Supervisors: Their place in Nursing, Midwifery & Health Visitor Education. Guidance letter, GL 2/92 Welsh National Board for Nursing, Midwifery & Health Visiting, Cardiff.

Woodrow, P. (1994) Mentorship: perceptions and pitfalls for nursing practice. *Journal of Advanced Nursing*, **19**, 812–8.

Chapter 5
Clinical Supervision and Reflective Practice

Introduction

Why include a chapter about clinical supervision in a book about reflective practice? Reflection is an activity which can be undertaken by oneself, however, engaging in critical reflection with another, as in clinical supervision, can have its advantages in extending personal interpretations to include other perspectives and viewpoints. Johns (1994), in the first edition of this book, called this 'guided reflection' and has since written much about this technique as a means of enabling practitioners to become more effective (e.g. Johns & Freshwater 1998). In this chapter the concept of clinical supervision will be described and the relationship with reflection will be explored with the aim of illustrating how the two processes can be utilised for the benefit of the individual practitioner, the organisation and the patient/client.

Background to the growth of clinical supervision in nursing

The 1990s have seen increasing attention paid to the concept of clinical supervision in nursing. This growth appears to be in response to two needs, one internal to the nursing profession and the other external:

- **internal** – recognition of the need to promote and develop professional practice and accountability
- **external** – the need to satisfy consumer demands by providing nursing care which maintains the safety of the client and adheres to a minimum standard.

Initial interest was fuelled by two important publications, 'A Vision for the Future' (DoH 1993) and a position paper on clinical supervision by Faugier & Butterworth (1994). This latter document was endorsed by the Chief Nursing Officer and was widely distributed for discussion with a view to the possible implementation of clinical supervision. Both of these publications came at a time when the development of professional practice, the safeguard of minimum standards of practice and the delivery of quality care were being promoted as essential to the maintenance of high standards of nursing practice and professional growth. The UKCC's (United Kingdom Central Council for Nursing, Midwifery and Health Visiting) statements on the guidelines for professional accountability (UKCC 1992a), post-registration education and practice – PREP (UKCC 1995) and the scope of professional practice (UKCC 1992b) were all highly significant in the promotion of autonomy and accountability in practice. These publications contributed to the perceived need for nurses constantly to evaluate their own performance and improve practice. The Clothier Report (DoH 1994) resulting from the Allitt enquiry further highlighted the need for good standards of supervision, training and education. The Allitt enquiry itself had raised the issue of professional standards in the minds of the general public, leading to an increased demand for professional regulation and supervision to safeguard the interests of the consumer. In this climate, clinical supervision soon became widely accepted as a means of providing support for nurses in the development of high quality practice while satisfying the concerns of the consumer.

My own interest in clinical supervision arises out of the potential it has for promoting personal and professional development of practitioners. Having worked for many years as a ward manager, I have a firm belief that the greatest asset of any team are the individual practitioners themselves. In my view, investing time and energy in each individual's professional growth, and helping practitioners to realise their own potential, pays dividends in the standards of care provided to the client as well as to the organisation as a whole. With increasing pressures of workload and the demands of the service, any activity which legitimises and facilitates this process is worthy of consideration.

What is clinical supervision?

Many authors have sought to define clinical supervision in a way that describes all aspects of the process, highlighting the positive outcomes for individual nurses as well as the quality of the nursing service. Clinical supervision has been described as:

'a term used to describe a formal process of professional support and learning which enables practitioners to develop knowledge and competence, assume responsibility for their own practice and enhance consumer protection and safety of care in complex situations.'

('A Vision for the Future', DoH 1993, p. 3)

The definition provided by Faugier & Butterworth is one that has been widely adopted as the simplest:

'an exchange between practising professionals to enable the development of professional skills.'

(Faugier & Butterworth 1994, p. 9)

Both of these definitions acknowledge the dynamic and formal nature of the process as a shared experience that enhances professional growth. The latter definition also provides a notion of a time frame for the supervisory activity, giving the impression that clinical supervision occurs within a focused discussion rather than as a continuous monitoring process. More recently, Bishop (1998a) has provided a definition that identifies other important components of clinical supervision, for example, the need for a safe and supportive environment in which clinical supervision may take place:

'Clinical supervision is a designated interaction between two or more practitioners, within a safe/supportive environment, which enables a continuum of reflective, critical analysis of care, to ensure quality patient services.'

(Bishop 1998a, p. 8)

In defining clinical supervision, the links with the process of reflection begin to emerge. Both processes claim to enable the practitioner to develop his or her professional knowledge, competence and skills through the analysis of practice. Furthermore, both are acknowledged as structured activities that occur within a certain framework. In some instances, the process of reflection is seen as a fundamental part of clinical supervision as in the definition provided by Bishop (1998a). There is also an acknowledgement that clinical supervision requires time, commitment and a safe and supportive environment for it to be most effective. These aspects are also fundamental to reflection as identified in other chapters of this book. The relationship between clinical supervision and reflection becomes even more visible as the aims and benefits of clinical supervision are considered.

Bishop (1994) identifies the most widely accepted aims of clinical supervision as being:

- a safeguard for standards of practice
- the development of professional expertise
- the delivery of quality care.

Proctor (1986) and Hawkins & Shohet (1989) describe three components of clinical supervision that provide a balanced view of the different ways in which it can be utilised. These are:

- **The formative or educative component:** This aims to develop the individual's skills, understanding and abilities.
- **The restorative or supportive component:** This provides emotional support for workers, helping them to understand their feelings about their therapeutic work with clients.
- **The normative or managerial component:** This aspect of clinical supervision provides an opportunity for quality control and the consideration of the organisational responsibilities of individuals.

The identified benefits of clinical supervision extend to the practitioner, the client, the profession and the organisation. Thus by discussing, analysing and evaluating practice, there is the potential for improvement in care as well as raised self awareness of the individual practitioner, increased effectiveness and professional growth and development. If this sounds familiar then it is because very similar claims are made of the process of reflection as explored throughout the chapters of this book.

The relationship between clinical supervision and reflection

Through consideration of the purpose and aims of clinical supervision it can be seen that reflection and clinical supervision are inextricably linked. Clinical supervision is sometimes seen as the formal and legitimate process by which practitioners can engage in reflection. An alternative view is that reflection is an essential component of clinical supervision.

The 'Vision for the Future' document suggested that clinical supervision was 'central to the process of learning and to the expansion of the scope of practice and should be seen as a means of encouraging self-assessment and analytical and reflective skills' (DoH 1993). Thus, the emphasis on learning through exploration and analysis of practice and self evaluation binds the processes of clinical supervision and reflection together. This view is shared by the UKCC (1996) who suggest that by encouraging reflection on practice issues, clinical supervision will enhance professional development and lifelong learning will be promoted.

Authors who have likened clinical supervision to the formal process in which practitioners can engage in reflection include Binnie & Titchen

(1995) who describe clinical supervision as a formal opportunity to informally discuss work with a colleague. These authors describe ways in which reflection can be utilised to develop understanding of practice and share expertise within a supervisory relationship. Fisher (1996) discusses the use of reflective practice in clinical supervision and suggests that the three components of clinical supervision – education, support and management – are also the focus of reflection and therefore, she argues, reflection enables clinical supervision. Similarly, Johns' (1994) and Johns & McCormack's (1998) work on guided reflection appears to suggest that this process is synonymous with clinical supervision. Johns' view is that reflection needs to be guided because practitioners require guidance to see beyond themselves and require the support and challenge to confront and resolve contradiction in everyday practice. Thus, as a formal process, guided reflection necessitates a relationship between a practitioner and a supervisor in a similar way to clinical supervision.

Within my own sphere of work, I have found that practitioners who understand and value the process of reflection often welcome the concept of clinical supervision as a way of formalising this activity. The benefits of utilising a reflective approach to practice may be transferred to a more formal structured process that provides further opportunities for practitioners to explore and analyse their practice. However, an important factor in the acceptance of clinical supervision as a similar process to reflection is the way in which it is set up in practice.

In implementing clinical supervision, it is recommended that practice units discuss and agree a practical understanding of the purpose, the process, the content and focus of clinical supervision and the relationship between supervision and management (Kohner 1994). This ensures that there is absolute clarity in the intention of clinical supervision and avoids potential conflict whereby it is seen purely as a management tool. In my own experience, I have found that clarification of this aspect of clinical supervision is crucial to its success. The inclusion of a managerial or normative aspect of clinical supervision often creates suspicions and anxieties in individual practitioners who fear that what is being introduced as a professional development tool may be utilised purely as a measure of job performance. It is interesting to note, however, that when practitioners are asked about the benefits of utilising reflection to explore and analyse their own practice, they often suggest that through development of their own skills and knowledge they will improve their own performance and thus hope to enhance patient care. These outcomes are very similar to those anticipated from the normative or management function of clinical supervision. The difference with reflection is that it is rarely implemented in such a formal way and is more usually seen as an activity that underpins the philosophy of a learning environment. Thus practitioners engage in reflection in a way which most appropriately suits their individual need for professional and practice development. In my view, the key to successful implementation of clinical supervision is to acknowledge the interrelationship between helping practitioners maximise their own potential and the potential for enhancement of the quality of care for patients. Seen from the viewpoint of the individual practitioner there is little conflict in these two aspects. Managers need to capitalise on this common aim and help practitioners recognise their own responsibility to the consumer rather than impose standards and performance indicators from above.

Although there may be some debate about the extent to which the reflective process is similar to clinical supervision, there is no doubt that the majority of the literature acknowledges that reflection plays an important role in the supervisory relationship. This is highlighted within the UKCC position paper on clinical supervision (1996, p. 4) in which key statement 2 states that clinical supervision is 'a practice-focused professional relationship involving a practitioner reflecting on practice guided by a skilled supervisor'. Even though this does rather assume that practitioners are familiar with the reflective process and that they have access to suitably skilled supervisors, it acknowledges the importance of reflective practice to the whole process. In different types of supervisory relationships, for example, one-to-one peer supervision and group supervision, reflection can also be a useful way of maintaining focus and ensuring the process of clinical supervision remains constructive.

In reviewing the efficacy of reflective practice within the context of clinical supervision, Fowler & Chevannes (1998) provide a counter argument and warn against an unquestioned acceptance that reflection is an integral part of the process. They suggest that while it is widely understood that clinical supervision is a way of harnessing reflective practice, it does not follow that clinical supervision should always utilise reflective practice. Their argument is that not all practitioners welcome the concept of reflection with its involvement of self and may find it unhelpful and alien to their way of thinking. This is a valid point in that practitioners who are unfamiliar with the use of reflection may find themselves inhibited by the process and thus may not engage in clinical supervision wholeheartedly. However, as it is clear that both the process of reflection and the process of clinical supervision require an element of self evaluation and self assessment, it is essential that individuals are encouraged and enabled to participate in this process. In circumstances where staff feel unwilling or unable to participate, for whatever reason, efforts must be made to address this before clinical supervision is implemented. This may entail exploring individuals' learning styles and examining the philosophy underpinning the local learning environment. As identified earlier, discussion and agreement about the purpose, process, content and focus of clinical supervision is essential for successful implementation.

Fowler & Chevannes (1998) also argue that for the person with little or no experience, reflection may be an inappropriate and frustrating method due to the lack of knowledge and experience to draw upon to make sense of practice. They suggest that more directive teaching may be more helpful in these circumstances. There is no doubt that one of the roles of the supervisor is to guide and perhaps direct the practitioner when a gap in knowledge or skill is identified, however, I do not feel that this precludes the individual from engaging in the reflective process. Many novice practitioners, including pre-registration students find the process of reflection rewarding and illuminating, as illustrated in this book. In trying to make sense of situations, the reflective process requires the individual to identify potential gaps in knowledge and search for new understandings by accessing appropriate resources. This may mean discussing the situation with a supervisor/mentor or accessing appropriate literature or raising to a conscious level knowledge which is embedded in practice but not yet visible.

The supervisory relationship

The success of clinical supervision relies to some extent on the quality and effectiveness of the supervisory relationship. In its guidelines for the introduction of clinical supervision, the Kings Fund states that it is essential that careful consideration is given to the qualifications, skills and experience required of supervisors, and to their ability to meet the individual needs of supervisees (Kohner 1994). However, in the first instance it is important to establish the nature of the supervisory relationship. This would include confirming the common purpose and beliefs about clinical supervision, agreeing appropriate ground rules to establish the boundaries of the supervisory relationship and the process of clinical supervision. This process needs to be entered into by all parties concerned. The individuals engaged in the supervision process will, of course, have a vested interest in ensuring there is agreement about the nature of the supervisory relationship. Similarly, the organisation will need to acknowledge the part it plays in determining this relationship. Providing opportunities for all parties to discuss and agree these aspects of clinical supervision may be the best way to avoid confusion about the purpose and the process of clinical supervision.

As mentioned earlier, it would appear from both the literature and my own experience that the greatest cause of anxiety about clinical supervision and the supervisory relationship is the emphasis placed on the managerial component. This has the potential to influence the nature of the supervision process, the choice of supervisor and the boundaries of the supervisory relationship. For example, can individuals choose their own supervisor? Does it always have to be someone more senior, or someone approved of by the manager? What part can group or peer supervision play? Who sets the agenda for each supervisory meeting?

Within the literature there is still some debate about the practicalities of implementing a clinical supervision process which combines professional support and growth with enhancement of the quality of services to clients (Burrow 1995). The UKCC (1996) has stated that clinical supervision is not the exercise of overt managerial responsibility or supervision, nor is it a system of formal individual performance review. Furthermore, it should not be considered hierarchical in nature. However, I believe that the role of the manager and the organisation is crucial in both of these aspects of clinical supervision. For example, while the individuals have a professional obligation to maintain their own personal and professional growth, they will achieve their objectives more successfully if they have the support of the manager and the organisation. Such support may include access to resources for further development or support in taking on new or different responsibilities or trying new ways of working. Similarly, the manager and organisation have a vested interest in establishing a workforce that is equipped to provide a quality service to clients. This often involves a commitment to support training and education and working to maximise the potential of each individual practitioner. In my view, discussion can reveal and highlight the similarities in these agendas rather than the potential conflicts.

One of the ways in which managers get to know the personal and professional aspirations of the practitioners within their workforce is through individual performance review. Kohner (1994) suggests that there can be links between clinical supervision and individual performance review. The implementation of such a system in which clinical supervision and performance review are linked has recently been described by Northcott (1998). He describes a contract between individuals and the organisation in which staff receive support and are nurtured as developing professionals, in exchange for the part they play in providing a high standard of care. The contract is discussed and agreed through individual performance review and the process is facilitated through clinical supervision. Potential conflict arising within this system is overcome by ensuring that control within the clinical supervision activity remains with the individual practitioner. Thus, while manager review is part of the performance review process, the individual practitioner decides upon his or her objectives and how these might be achieved through clinical supervision. It would appear that an important aspect of this process is that the individual feels comfortable with the supervisory relationship and has the opportunity to influence the choice of supervisor. Northcott (1998) describes how this is agreed upon through discussion and exploration of the most appropriate method of supervision and the most appropriate supervisor. Again, a key element here is willingness to discuss the process in an open and honest manner, acknowledging the viewpoints of all parties concerned.

There will be organisations in which, for whatever reason there is a lack of openness and a lack of willingness to address these issues in a collaborative way. In these circumstances it may be more beneficial for clinical supervision to be utilised for its formative/educative and restorative/supportive components with less emphasis on its normative/ managerial component. This would allow engagement in the process while minimising the potential for conflict. This viewpoint is supported by Carthy (1994) who suggests that performance supervision that includes topics such as communication, teamwork, attitudes, innovative practice and communicating organisational initiatives, is best carried out by line managers. Thus, this is seen here as being quite different from clinical supervision.

The nature of the supervisory relationship is further explored by Johns & McCormack (1998) who liken the therapeutic relationship between supervisor and practitioner to that of the client and practitioner. They state that the central role of the supervisor is to work with the practitioner towards achieving their best interests just as the practitioner works with the client to achieve a similar goal. In order to achieve this, Johns & McCormack (1998) suggest that the supervisor and practitioner are required to share a similar vision of clinical practice and supervision. This is not to say that they have to agree on everything but if there is an imbalance in the perceived intent or emphasis of clinical supervision then it is unlikely that the potential for achievement will be realised. Thus if the supervisees perceive that the intent of clinical supervision is to judge their performance, they may be less likely to disclose information about their practice experiences. This suggests that the 'comfort zone', that is, the climate of trust and openness, required for clinical supervision is an essential element of the supervisory relationship. In order to achieve constructive self assessment and self evaluation, which includes the opportunity to question practice, a safe and supportive environment is required. This very much echoes some of the pre-requisites for reflective practice. It also lends some credence to the notion that the supervisee should have some say in the choice of supervisor.

Goorapah (1997) states that there may be a potential conflict in the roles of supervisor and supporter which is not dissimilar to the conflict sometimes experienced by the mentor who acts as supporter and assessor at the same time. He suggests that the problem is compounded if the supervisor is also the manager of the supervisee. It could be argued that when the supervisor is the manager, greater care must be taken to avoid the abuse of the position of power invested in the management role. There is also the danger of conflicting agendas, unwillingness to take on new ideas which conflict with management processes, and the potential for fostering dependence in supervisees rather than empowering them in their clinical autonomy. However, the manager also has a unique insight into the practice of the supervisee, he or she may be able to facilitate the achievement of specific goals and may combine the work of supervision and growth of the individual with the growth of the organisation.

In all supervisory relationships, particularly those in which the manager is the supervisor, it is essential that ground rules are agreed to establish the boundaries of the relationship. Kohner (1994) suggests that it is helpful if individual and mutual responsibilities are agreed at the start and expectations recorded. As with other types of supervisory relationships, ground rules can establish codes of conduct relating to confidentiality, respect for individual viewpoints and terms of contact. It is especially important to clarify expectations with respect to the latter point, the type and length of contact. Clinical supervision rarely involves constant monitoring of an individual's performance and more often involves meeting together for a set period of time to discuss practice. Supervisory meetings can involve the individual supervisor and supervisee or may include group supervision. It would therefore be useful to agree in advance when and where to meet, how often and for how long and who should be involved. The structure and focus of supervisory sessions can also be discussed and agreed upon, including the part reflection plays in the process.

It is within these types of supervisory relationships that reflection plays an important role in the clinical supervision process. The use of a reflective framework facilitates a structured approach to the agenda of the supervisory meeting and helps to maintain the focus on practice while enabling a questioning approach. The knowledge, skills and attitudes important to reflective practice will also be important here and will become part of the ground rules of the relationship.

The role of supervisor

The role of the supervisor in clinical supervision is not dissimilar to the role of mentor or preceptor although it is generally agreed that the latter two terms are more frequently applied to novice or new practitioners who require educational input and support (Faugier & Butterworth 1994). Much has been written about the mentor role that is useful in consideration of the role of the clinical supervisor. For example, the Darling MMP – Measuring Mentoring Potential (Darling 1984) describes some of the essential characteristics of the ideal mentor which include both interpersonal skills and reflective skills useful in all helping relationships. Similarly, the characteristics of the reflective mentor are identified in Brigid Reid's chapter, Chapter 4, within this book.

Many authors have attempted to describe the essential features of the role of the clinical supervisor. For example, Faugier (1992) presents a growth and support model of supervision acknowledging that the role of the supervisor is to facilitate growth both educationally and personally in the supervisee, while providing essential support to their clinical autonomy. Faugier & Butterworth (1994) adapt a model derived from Frankham (1987) to describe the functions of the supervisor and Johns and McCormack (1998) explore the conditions for an effective supervisory relationship.

In reviewing the literature relating to the role of clinical supervisor, it becomes clear that some of the most important aspects of the role are the attributes and attitudes displayed by the individual supervisors and their willingness to facilitate learning in others, while employing a reflective and questioning approach to their own role. Clinical supervisors should be willing to:

- take on the role and engage in negotiations regarding the process and focus of clinical supervision
- commit time and energy to clinical supervision activities
- listen to the individual being supervised and acknowledge their agenda for learning
- use reflection and questioning techniques to explore the individual practitioner's understanding of practice
- explore new ideas, share their own experiences and be willing to be thought-provoking
- provide support and challenge to enhance development in the practitioner
- engage in the process with sensitivity, acknowledging the need for confidentiality and the promotion of mutual trust

● undertake training and preparation and engage in clinical supervision themselves.

It is generally agreed that all supervisors should be given the opportunity to receive training and preparation to take on their role (UKCC 1996) and that all supervisors should engage in clinical supervision themselves (Kohner 1994). This latter point is extremely important in that it not only informs the supervisor about the experience of clinical supervision but it provides an opportunity for them to reflect upon their own role and receive appropriate support and supervision themselves. It also promotes engagement in the clinical supervision process at all levels within the organisation as all those who provide supervision will necessarily be given supervision themselves. The establishment of such a structure may be extremely helpful in ensuring that the outcomes of clinical supervision are realised at all levels. However, the potential difficulties of ensuring such a system operates should not be underestimated. It is often the most senior nurses who lack the opportunity to engage in activities such as clinical supervision or reflective practice. This may be for a number of reasons including lack of suitable supervisors, lack of time or lack of commitment.

As Scanlon (1998) points out, it is unfortunate that there is little guidance with regard to the level and kind of training which should be made available to clinical supervisors. The UKCC have chosen not to be prescriptive in this respect and have left it up to Trusts to decide upon local training needs. While this provides an opportunity for Trusts to mould the supervision training to their own processes, it does rely on the relative importance each Trust places on this aspect of clinical supervision. The current climate within the NHS has tended to ensure that there is fierce competition for resources linked with training and education and thus to be successful, clinical supervision and the requirements for training will need to be supported at the highest level.

Interestingly, Fowler (1996) states that many of the skills required for a supervisor, for example, negotiation, interpersonal and coaching skills and the facilitation of self evaluation can be equated with equivalent patient care skills. Therefore, he suggests that it may be unnecessary to have a complete training programme on supervision if the transfer of established skills from patient care to clinical supervision is facilitated. This view accords with that of Johns & McCormack (1998) who highlight the similarities between the supervisory relationship and the practitioner/client relationship. To some extent, there appears to be an assumption here that nurse–client relationships are well developed, that all those practitioners who may engage in clinical supervision will have highly developed patient care skills and that they will be able to transfer these skills to the supervisory relationship easily.

Those practitioners who are considering taking on the role of clinical supervisor may find it useful to reflect upon their own attitudes towards the process of clinical supervision and their willingness to fulfil the supervisory role. As mentioned earlier, an essential component of clinical supervision is the willingness to undertake self assessment and evaluation. This is not dissimilar to the pre-requisites for reflective practice and practitioners may find it helpful to begin by ensuring that they are familiar and comfortable with this process. It would also be useful for practitioners to consider the strengths they have to contribute to the role of supervisor, identifying any transferable skills that they may utilise in other situations (for example, in client interactions or in mentor roles) and analysing their potential usefulness to the supervisory role.

The role of the supervisee

One can argue that many of the characteristics required of individuals engaging in reflective practice hold true for those engaging in clinical supervision. In order to get the most out of clinical supervision, individual practitioners must be willing to embrace the process with a degree of honesty and openness. There should be a commitment to self enquiry and a readiness to change practice.

Supervisees are encouraged to be proactive within the supervisory relationship (Hawkins & Shohet 1989), ensuring that they get the supervision they want by taking full responsibility for the part they play in negotiating the supervision contract. Supervisees need to recognise that they have an equal role in monitoring and evaluating the supervisory relationship (Kohner 1994). Ground rules to establish boundaries within the supervisory relationship need to be set jointly.

Proctor (1988, cited in Hawkins & Shohet 1989) provides guidelines for supervisees to help them realise their responsibilities. These are:

- identify practice issues with which you need help and ask for help
- become increasingly able to share freely
- identify what responses you want
- become more aware of the organisational contracts that affect supervisor, clients and supervisee
- be open to feedback
- monitor tendencies to justify, explain or defend
- develop the ability to discriminate what feedback is useful.

While these guidelines may just as easily be applied to the student in the mentor–student relationship, it should be remembered that in this circumstance, the supervisee is a qualified practitioner who should expect to take some responsibility for their own professional development.

Johns (1994) in describing the supervision phase of his model for guided reflection suggests that the practitioner reflect upon practice incidents before the supervision session in order to utilise supervision time for more critical reflection. This requires a commitment on behalf of the supervisee to prepare for supervision sessions in order to make best use of them. One way of achieving this is to keep a reflective diary. This has advantages in that it enables the practitioner to pick and choose from appropriate learning incidents as well as reviewing the learning that has taken place over time. It also ensures that the practitioner remains in control of the supervision agenda (as discussed earlier).

In considering participation in the supervision process it would be just as pertinent for practitioners to reflect upon their attitudes towards clinical supervision as it is for the supervisors. To realise the potential of clinical supervision, practitioners should consider what they want to get out of the activity, what sort of supervision they require and how they might best prepare to embark on the supervisory process. Using a reflective approach in everyday practice may be a first step to opening the door to effective clinical supervision.

The reality of clinical supervision in practice

One would think that considering the endorsement received for clinical supervision from policy makers and nursing leaders, the practice of clinical supervision would be well established, however, this is not so. In her survey of Trusts within Scotland and England, with a response rate of 67%, Bishop (1998c) identified that the majority of respondents were engaged in some form of clinical supervision. Many of these had only just implemented clinical supervision (mean 2.5 years in the community and 9 months in the acute sector) or clinical supervision was only partially implemented across the Trust. The key problems identified by the questionnaire in the implementation of clinical supervision were:

- an ever-increasing workload
- money for staff time and staff training
- management and staff perceptions
- training options and facilities for supervisors.

It is evident that the implementation of clinical supervision requires managerial commitment at all levels of the organisation in order to overcome some of the other difficulties. Furthermore, it also requires the commitment of the individual practitioners to engage in supervisory relationships. In the NHS of the late 1990s, with its resource and staffing problems, it is difficult to suggest to overburdened staff that they must find time to engage in such activities. However, there is evidence to suggest that it is these very activities which provide support for individual practitioners, helping to reduce stress and burnout. Kohner (1994) states that clinical supervision is an investment in staff and that it acknowledges and affirms the value of nurses and nursing. Bishop's survey (1998c) identifies support and valuing staff; improved staff morale; increased staff commitment; a reduction in sickness rates, improved recruitment and retention and reduced stress levels as some of the key perceived or evaluated benefits of clinical supervision.

In order to consider the benefits and possibilities of clinical supervision to you and your organisation and to help you consider what you can do to promote clinical supervision within your own unit, consider the following questions:

- What support systems do you have in place within your unit and how effective are they?
- Is stress recognised and dealt with within your unit? If so, what coping strategies are employed and how effective are they?
- How often do you share your thoughts and experiences of nursing with others and how productive is this?
- How do you learn in practice? Have you set yourself learning objectives?
- How do you know that you are achieving your goals?
- Do you and your colleagues engage in reflective practice?
- Have you ever given or received supervision? How did it feel? Was it useful?
- Could you utilise reflection as a means of providing support and supervision to each other?
- What reasons do you have for not engaging in reflection or clinical supervision? Examine each of these to try to find positive solutions.
- What can you offer as a clinical supervisor?

Conclusion

This chapter has discussed the relationship between reflection and clinical supervision and has established that there are considerable similarities in the aims and outcomes of the two processes. Clinical supervision can be seen as a way of utilising reflective practice not only to enhance individual performance and self awareness but also to achieve organisational aims of maintenance of standards of care and an improved quality of service. Furthermore, the potential for increased levels of support, motivation and morale when engaging in reflective practice with another can be further realised through the adoption of clinical supervision.

There are, however, a number of factors that may influence the successful implementation of clinical supervision. One such factor is the willingness of organisations to embrace the concept of clinical supervision and to mobilise the necessary resources to ensure its success. In the present climate within the NHS it is tempting to ignore any activity which does not provide immediate benefits or whose outcomes cannot be easily measured. Clinical supervision may be a casualty of this. It will require determination from nurse leaders to ensure that approaches such as clinical supervision and reflective practice are supported in order that their potential long-term benefits may be realised. It may also require a willingness to look beyond the purely quantitative methods of evaluation. This is clearly an area that requires further research and discussion.

Another important factor in the successful implementation of clinical supervision is the willingness of practitioners to engage in this process themselves. This willingness must go beyond a positive endorsement of the concept. The challenge for practitioners is to find the necessary time and energy to invest in their own and others' personal and professional growth, to see it as important and to do something about it. This may mean canvassing managers for their support and engaging in discussion about the aims and purpose of the process but it may also mean giving something of oneself to ensure its successful implementation. I would encourage all practitioners to ask themselves what part clinical supervision and reflective practice has to play in their professional lives and how they wish to see the future of nursing. As potential leaders of the future, it is the decisions made by today's practitioners that will be important. This will be the major influence in deciding whether clinical supervision and reflective practice are just another trendy phase or become an established part of nursing practice.

References and further reading

Binnie, A. & Titchen, A. (1995) The art of clinical supervision. *British Journal of Nursing*, **4**, 327–34.

Bishop, V. (1994) Clinical supervision for an accountable profession. *Nursing Times*, **90** (39), 35–7.

Bishop, V. (1998a) Clinical supervision: what is it? In Bishop, V. (ed) *Clinical Supervision in Practice*, Macmillan/NT Research, London, pp. 1–2.

Bishop, V. (ed) (1998b) *Clinical Supervision in Practice*, Macmillan/NT Research, London.

Bishop, V. (1998c) Clinical supervision: what is going on? Results of a questionnaire. *NT Research*, **3** (2), 141–50.

Burrow, S. (1995) Supervision: clinical development or management control? *British Journal of Nursing*, **4**, 879–82.

Carthy, J. (1994) Bandwagons roll. *Nursing Standard*, **8** (38), 48–9.

Darling, L. (1984) What do nurses want in a mentor? *Journal of Nursing Administration*, **14** (10), 42–4.

Department of Health (1993) *A Vision for the Future: The Nursing, Midwifery and Health Visiting Contribution to Health and Health Care*, HMSO, London.

Department of Health (1994) *The Allitt Inquiry*, (The Clothier Report). HMSO, London.

Faugier, J. (1992) The supervisory relationship. In Butterworth, T. & Faugier, J. *Clinical Supervision and Mentorship in Nursing*, pp.18–36. Chapman & Hall, London.

Faugier, J. & Butterworth, T. (1994) *Clinical Supervision: A Position Paper*, University of Manchester, Manchester.

Fisher, M. (1996) Using reflective practice in clinical supervision. *Professional Nurse*, **11** (7), 443–4.

Fowler, J. (1996) The organisation of clinical supervision within the nursing profession: a review of the literature. *Journal of Advanced Nursing*, **23**, 471–8.

Fowler, J. & Chevannes, M. (1998) Evaluating the efficacy of reflective practice within the context of clinical supervision. *Journal of Advanced Nursing*, **27**, 379–82.

Goorapah, D. (1997) Clinical supervision. *Journal of Clinical Nursing*, **6**, 173–8.

Hawkins, P. & Shohet, R. (1989) *Supervision in the Helping Professions*, Open University Press, Buckingham.

Johns, C. (1994) Guided reflection. In Palmer, A., Burns, S. & Bulman, C. (eds) *Reflective Practice in Nursing*, Blackwell Scientific Publications, Oxford, pp. 110–130.

Johns, C. & Freshwater, D. (eds) (1998) *Transforming Nursing Through Reflective Practice*, Blackwell Science, Oxford.

Johns, C. & McCormack, B. (1998) Illuminating the transformative potential of guided reflection. In Johns, C. & Freshwater, D. (eds) *Transforming Nursing Through Reflective Practice*, Blackwell Science, Oxford, pp. 78–90.

Kohner, N. (1994) *Clinical Supervision in Practice*, Kings Fund Centre, London.

Northcott, N. (1998) The development of guidelines on clinical supervision in clinical practice settings. In Bishop, V. (ed) *Clinical Supervision in Practice*, Macmillan/NT Research, London, pp. 109–142.

Proctor, B. (1986) Supervision: a co-operative exercise in accountability. In Marken, M. & Payne, M. (eds) *Enabling and Ensuring*, Leicester National

Youth Bureau and Council for Education and Training in Youth and Community Work.

Scanlon, C. (1998) Towards effective training of clinical supervisors. In Bishop, V. (ed) *Clinical Supervision in Practice*, Macmillan/NT Research, London, pp. 143–62.

United Kingdom Central Council for Nursing, Midwifery & Health Visiting (1992a) *Code of Conduct for the Nurse, Midwife and Health Visitor*, UKCC, London.

United Kingdom Central Council for Nursing, Midwifery & Health Visiting (1992b) *The Scope of Professional Practice*, UKCC, London.

United Kingdom Central Council for Nursing, Midwifery & Health Visiting (1995) *Standards for Post-Registration Education and Practice (PREP)*, UKCC, London.

United Kingdom Central Council for Nursing, Midwifery & Health Visiting (1996) *Position Statement on Clinical Supervision for Nursing and Health Visiting*, UKCC, London.

Chapter 6
Students' Perspectives on Reflective Practice

Introduction

'Are you feeling confounded by reflection and overawed by adult and self directed learning?'

(Holm & Stephenson 1994, p. 53)

So opened the student's chapter in the first edition of this book. Five years on have these feelings of uncertainty changed? Certainly there has been an increase in the use of reflection as nurse education seeks to find a tool that can enhance the development of thinking, questioning practitioners. Consequently there exist a greater number of mentors and practitioners who have experienced reflective learning processes for themselves, and this number must have its influence on the experiences of today's students. We felt it important therefore to take another look at the student perspective on reflection.

In updating this chapter the editors again decided to go 'to the horse's mouth' and obtain the views of nurses currently undertaking nurse education where reflection is key to the learning process. It was felt that these participants would have experiences that were worth sharing with other students starting out on a process of reflection, as well as with educationalists, and that these would build on the student's experiences expressed in the first edition.

A focus group was used to produce qualitative data in order to provide insights into the attitudes, perceptions and opinions of the participants (McElroy 1997, Basch 1987).

A group of nurses, who were mature, post-registration palliative care diploma and degree students, were invited to a discussion facilitated by the authors. In order to prepare the participants for the discussion a list of questions was drawn up to give focus to the discussion and to provide a clearly identifiable agenda. The questions reflected the concerns of the students who wrote in the first edition of this book; these included:

- What does reflection mean to you?
- How do you think your previous educational experiences have influenced your way of learning?
- How was the process of reflection introduced to you?
- What are your feelings about the way that reflection was introduced to you?
- Can you tell us about your early experiences of using reflection?
- What sort of factors influenced your ability to keep on developing your reflection?
- What sort of practical things helped you to develop a reflective piece of work?
- How do you reflect now? What strategies do you use? Who do you reflect with?
- Do you feel that reflection has worked for you as a tool for learning?

We were hopeful of getting a free flowing discussion whereby ideas and issues were responded to openly between group members. Permission was gained to tape the focus group meeting, rather than rely on note taking throughout the discussion; this allowed the facilitators to create a more relaxed and spontaneous environment. The participants did relax as they got into the discussion and were enthusiastic to share their experiences with us, prompted by our questions. The tapes produced were transcribed and the transcriptions analysed separately by each author and then jointly in order to explore themes relating to the attitudes, perceptions and opinions of the participants.

Themes

In reviewing the themes the authors felt it was important to use a framework to organise and coherently present the experiences collected from the focus group. We chose a time-related continuum as the information generally followed the progress of the students using reflection in their course of study and clinical practice. It also seemed logical; however some points raised in one section may have relevance in another.

The findings are divided into three areas:

(1) **Starting out** – the period when reflection is introduced. Getting going with first efforts and how that feels.
(2) **Gaining experience** – keeping motivated and how to take the work to a deeper level.
(3) **Moving on** – what happens after the focus of learning passes and

you are left with some level of reflective skills? What are you going to do with these skills?

Practical tips

From each of these areas we were also able to identify practical tips for the novice reflector, these are presented in Table 6.1 at the end of the chapter. We hope that these will prove useful as a quick reference point for those of you tackling reflection for the first time or for the educationalist considering developing students' reflective abilities.

Starting out

On starting out it was evident that the way the tutor formally introduced reflection to the students was important. At the beginning of their course students experienced a teaching session which helped to clarify their knowledge and experience, allowing them to test their understanding and begin to explore this new notion of reflection.

> 'We had a lot of support initially in a question and answer format in case we didn't understand it (reflection). Obviously we were given lots of references as well that we could go away and read so that we would feel more comfortable with it. I think until you have a go at it you never learn how to do it, there's no right or wrong way to start. . . .I think it was the support really that made it a bit easier.'

Support and guidance are noted as important within the literature (Daloz 1986) if prospective reflective practitioners are to be able to open up to new ways of looking at their practice. Support and guidance are also necessary in order to survive the challenge that reflection may create to a practitioner's present practice, since it may expose the need to confront uncomfortable and difficult issues concerning the individual and his or her practice environment. In addition there is a need to give students academic guidance about how to use and develop the reflective process (Burrows 1995, Johns 1995, Paterson 1995). In this case as well as exploring the students' own understanding the tutor clearly explained the academic expectations, and how the reflective process fitted in. The key people involved in this were identified as the students themselves, their mentor, their tutor and their student colleagues. This process began to allay some of the concerns of those students unfamiliar with reflection. The theoretical explanation of the reflective cycle, (Gibbs 1988) see Figure 4.2, was also valued as something concrete to hold on to and refer to while in the process.

The hurdle of actually getting something down on paper was commented on strongly. Students began to realise the impact of actually writing down thoughts; things previously 'just in the mind', and how in some way, writing them down substantiated and, perhaps, subtly changed their thoughts. Students also commented that writing down private thoughts on paper moved them from the private to the public domain and thus opened them up to scrutiny in ways unfamiliar and potentially uncomfortable. They expressed the need to feel safe when sharing their early work with mentors and tutors. While some students felt uncomfortable handing in what they viewed as unfinished work, others were happy to hand in work that could be developed further following discussion with their tutor/mentor.

'One of the things that I find difficult about the assignments and the reflective learning contract business, is that the way I like to learn and study is to write something and reflect on that and then to leave it, and for me personally to sit on it. This business of having to get it to my supervisor, for her to feedback before it was finished I have not liked. To try and present a half-finished piece of work is not the way that I like to be. I like to have it sorted in my head. I don't like sharing half baked ideas.'

'I was completely different once I got the hang of it. I think because my mentor was very experienced in the whole learning contract business. I felt like, he knows what he's doing so he won't let me go far wrong. So I was quite happy to splurge a bit and give him some of my reflections. I thought it's not like I'm giving the whole thing in. . . . I could give in a half baked piece of work and he'd come back and say this is half baked, so I was quite happy.'

This seems to demonstrate that for some students the way that the formal process of reflective work is organised within the educational system may be uncomfortable. The literature certainly has words of warning with regard to students' written reflection, which requires sharing with the teacher. It may increase a sense of powerlessness in relation to their practice area and students may find the laborious business of writing in journal form a difficult task to keep going (Wellard & Bethune 1996, Paterson 1995). However current thinking suggests that developing writing ability is not just a way of recording thought but is also a way to develop thinking and that this necessarily has a positive effect on nurses' practice development (Allen *et al.* 1989, Heinrich 1992).

The students increasingly appreciated the impact of their previous learning. Their experiences of a didactic approach to learning at school, in nurse training and at university influenced their acceptance of the validity of knowledge from those in positions of status and authority.

'When I was at university the great and the good professor somebody or other would have written about whatever theory it was. At 18 you assume that he knows a lot about everything, then as time goes on you think, wait a minute this person is nearly the same age as me! Perhaps actually, I don't need to take what they say as gospel.'

'As an older student I have found it very difficult to be critical of the written word. To me you know if it was written down, the good and the great wrote it down, and so you didn't question and I think I'm still struggling with that.'

'I trained a very long time ago, and then it was so and so says this in a textbook. Your assignments that you did during your training were very much case studies, it was either I did this or I did that and as long as you knew you had done it in the right order it was ok. No one asked you to reflect on whether it was right! There was a sort of tick list like laying up a trolley.'

Some comment was made to the effect that some personalities may find reflection easier to do and that this was not necessarily tied up with previous learning experiences.

'I think there are some people who find reflection easy and some people that don't. I think that comes down partly to personality. There are some people who will always mull things over . . . some people who would not consider an event ever again.'

It is strongly evident in the literature that reflective skills are not easy to develop and that the challenge that is created in terms of examination of one's close beliefs may mean that reflection is not comfortable. This seems to be something that should be carefully noted by educationalists despite the message that reflective skills can indeed be taught (Burrows 1995, James & Clarke 1994, Paterson 1995, Hargreaves 1997).

Anxieties about lack of nursing experience at the beginning of the process were evident. This was focused for these students, for example, on the lack of recent care of dying patients while studying a module about death and dying. There were concerns that they would have nothing to reflect upon. It is important to mention the work of Schön (1991) here who believes that practitioners build up a repertoire of practice experiences and knowledge that can be applied to new situations. This has important implications for those educating and supporting students with little or no experience of nursing to draw upon, particularly when the anxieties of experienced nurses such as those in this focus group are evident. These feelings are echoed in the reflections of Holm and Stephenson:

'Trying very hard to get down to my learning contract and reflection, I am getting very, very stressed. I don't know what I'm expected to be reflecting on, I cannot see how I can achieve the competencies let alone prove that I have achieved them ... I want to do well and I want to be able to assert myself enough so that I can help myself to do well.'

Holm & Stephenson (1994) p55.

There are also concerns in the literature as to whether young adults are able to think in a reflective way. Burrows (1995) cites some interesting research studies focusing on the subject. These concerns apply to the typical college age student and are relevant in relation to the average nursing student trying to grapple with reflection, particularly when one notes the difficulties expressed by the mature students above, who according to the research are presumably cognitively prepared to take on reflection.

The students felt it was important to get something down on paper and this seemed to be one of the most important hurdles to get over. This appeared to describe their own struggles in developing their critical abilities. They devised ways of handling this, for example they needed to stand back from what they had written in order to begin to be critical. This meant leaving what they had written for a couple of days in order to get a better perspective on it.

'I write something and then go away and leave it, I did find it helped to do that, because I find that I get so close to it that I couldn't make any judgements about whether it was any good. I'd spend one or two paragraphs thinking that this is a cracker and six hours later think this is absolute garbage. I couldn't get a perspective on it until I went away, and then when I came back and had given it some more thought I could easily pare away, ... this is superfluous, cut this; that really helped.'

'I remember doing a very small piece of work. I thought I'm probably not going to include this in my learning contract. Actually in the end, I did include it in the piece of work, with a squiggled note saying this is an idea, I hope it is all right. I found it very useful just to give myself permission to do something, which I wasn't going to include as a sort of practice item to start with and then going back to my mentor. ... Just give yourself permission to do a little bit of practice. Not something that is terribly academic either, get the idea of the Gibbs cycle and how to do that before you go into the learning contract.'

Over and above this, discussion with their tutor/mentor and other students was key in taking this further. They also found reading about reflection in the literature and seeking cues from other academic work useful. At this point they were beginning to get to grips with the other processes involved such as reflective learning contracts and to use them in their own way to capitalise on their own learning style.

The end of the starting out period was marked by the realisation that reflection was merely a tool for learning and can be managed and manoeuvred by the student and not something which is put on a pedestal and thought to be more than it is.

> 'Sometimes there is this impression that it is more than it is (reflection), but you've got to keep reminding yourself that it is a tool, a tool for learning and it might be that it is not necessarily the right tool for you, as a learner, in that we all have different ways of learning.'

Gaining experience

While in the midst of a course of study or learning, keeping motivated is important. Reflection seemed to help these students keep motivated because it was related to their practice. Consequently day-to-day work was more enjoyable and students seemed to feel more focused and effective in their practice because they had a strategy that helped them to deal with the realities of their daily work. Motivation was also stimulated by the educationalists who provided different creative and enjoyable ways for the students to develop the reflective process.

> 'I think that the course has been particularly good in getting us to use reflection a different way and that's made it more enjoyable, the different ways we've used it throughout the course.'

The coaching abilities of the tutor seemed to be very important. This involved giving balanced feedback, getting students to question things, being non-judgemental as well as being human enough to share his or her own vulnerability and mistakes. However there were mixed views about how students felt as they developed a relationship with the tutor over time.

> 'I think that Janice [the tutor] was very good at giving a balanced argument on both sides with regard to anything we were learning about, so she tried to get you to question things. I think she came across therefore in a non-judgemental way.'

> 'she was very human, she was able to share her own vulnerability and mistakes that she'd made and the things that she'd gaffed over, so you knew that she hadn't put herself on a pedestal and in my eyes was just normal.'

> 'I seemed to have no problem about waffling on about the way that I feel. I found it difficult – I found it worse actually laying myself open, until I knew the tutor.'

'She (the tutor) is brilliant at feedback I have to say and sometimes there is a little bit of humour in what she says, but still taking you forward all the time.'

It is interesting to note that the trustworthiness, quality and quantity of feedback and the coaching abilities of the teacher are deemed important in the literature, having a major impact on the students' ability and willingness to reflect (Schön 1991, Paterson 1995, Carr 1996). Also demonstrated here is an appreciation of the adult-centred approach of the teacher thought to be instrumental in the development of reflective, critical practitioners (French & Cross 1992). It is also evident here that the tutor had a reflective and enquiry-orientated approach.

The ongoing support of the mentor was also a key factor in gaining experience. Students commented on the mixed abilities of the mentors to help them. The preparation of mentors and their experience both of nursing and mentoring seemed to be significant. The students appeared to have very high expectations of their mentors, for example expecting them to have a high academic achievement and extensive clinical experience. However, this was tempered by a reluctant realisation that the ideal may be difficult to achieve in the current climate.

A good experience seemed to rely on the mentor knowing what was expected of the student, being confident of reflection themselves, and being able to challenge the student to 'move up a gear' to achieve a more academic level. Reflection thereby moves from a reflective conversation between student and mentor to a process where the student has analysed related literature and further experience, in order to complete the reflective cycle. There appeared to be an increasing sense of becoming familiar with the process of reflection.

'I think once you've started it's something that becomes natural, more natural to do...'

There was also an appreciation of the fact that this type of learning was related to practice, this was something the students could relate to in a positive way. There was evidence that students discussed their work and learnt from each other in their attempts to deepen their levels of reflection.

'Being practice related has helped very much and just something that is quite small can make a big difference... I can remember you saying [referring to another student] "just remember to go deep rather than wide", because it was such a clear image in my mind, and I went on from there really.'

Students began to see the relevance of the reflective process in their academic work and in their practice. There was a realisation that reflection was not a rigid template to be applied uniformly, and students adapted the process to meet their own learning needs. Students appreciated the chance to self evaluate at the end of each piece of reflective work. They had a sense of direction for their future learning.

> 'I think the other thing that we're encouraged to do ... is think where are we, where are we going ... I think that helps to realise that there are still things that you need to explore, so it is ongoing'

Moving on

Even though the students had come to the end of their programmes of study, they felt they would continue to reflect. They continued to use reflection in an informal way even though they were not jumping through the hoops of academic assignments.

> 'I suppose mentally it's still there [Gibbs cycle]. I had to do this personal statement for the profile in a reflective way. I didn't have it structured so much with the cycle but I did have it in mind, that's stuck with me.'

The students seemed to be using their reflective experience to deal with things but on looking back were not always aware that they were formally using it. In this sense there was a feeling that academic study had influenced their practice. They pointed out that in order to be a professional practitioner it is important to analyse what you are doing, and the students viewed the reflective process as a way to achieve this. It was described as a process of enrichment. Interestingly they found it hard to describe what it was like before they started using the process. There was a sense that they needed to find like minded colleagues or friends to maintain and develop their reflective skills.

> 'One of my colleagues recently went on maternity leave but reflection was something that we did on a regular basis. After every patient we would just talk about the patient and then deeper issues were brought up, we'd just air them between ourselves. Whereas now I'm working with a colleague, she is definitely not into reflecting, not even chatting so much, she just gets on with her work and I find it quite difficult. I'm really missing the discussions about patients ... I'm going to have to be careful I don't lose the skill.'

There was an appreciation that the pace of the working environment was important in finding time for reflection. If they were in a busy environment they would need to structure it in.

'I remember where I worked before, the place was just so frantic all the time that there was no opportunity to reflect at all, actually there was never a minute, there were people badgering me about things all the time. Working in the community this is easier, you've got ten minutes in the car to think about what happened before you get to the next person. So in some situations it would need to be more formal where you actually need to sit down together and work out why a situation was so disastrous. I would like to think that you would never not do that'.

It appeared that reflection had enabled students to recognise their own personal learning style, which was something that did not happen for some of them in past educational experiences. Generally they expressed a greater level of confidence and a more critical approach to academic work and the ability to challenge things more in practice. There was a general awareness of the transferability of reflective skills too, for example, clinical supervision and profiling. Interestingly, Johns (1995) would say that clinical supervision is the key to unlocking this reflective potential further and he discusses the value of this for nursing in his work.

Students commented on development of self: self awareness, self empowerment, self confidence, self control, and being more able to challenge and be critical. Reflection seemed to have challenged some set ideas, and established feelings of being more open.

'It's definitely made me question the way I behave in front of patients. The way I communicate with them and sometimes my feelings about things afterwards: to be more non-judgemental, to question everything.'

'I try to see things from other people's points of view instead of just being critical, in terms of a negative idea of a colleague's behaviour.'

There was a greater awareness of the impact students had on other people and there was a sense that they could stand back and analyse other's reactions towards themselves, and that this might lead to a different outcome. It was also noted that they could see others' points of view.

'the impact you have on others and the effect you have, I found that quite a learning curve.'

'it's all about challenging yourself; why am I doing this? why did I think that? why am I not doing this?'

'I have found it very useful at times to think well I wonder why that person is reacting in that way and instead of reacting to them immediately, standing back and thinking about it and analysing it, and then doing something completely different from what I would have initially done. So I found it (reflection) really, really useful in that respect. I found it quite comforting I suppose really. In a way, I suppose it can make you... I want to say more powerful, I don't really mean powerful I suppose I mean more self confident.'

Conclusion

Presenting the student's perspective through a focus group has enabled us to share the experiences of a number of students with the reader. By using the concerns raised by Stephenson and Holm in the first edition of this book as the basis for our questions with this focus group, we have been able to check out the relevance of these concerns five years on. While one must be aware of the biases with this form of enquiry, it may be that the reader will recognise these concerns and this may serve to validate them, in terms of your own personal experience.

It is true that several key educational theorists propose the concept of reflection as a tool for learning and indeed have analysed the processes of reflection (Boud *et al.* 1985, Van Manen 1977, Mezirow 1981, Schön 1991). However there is no doubt that extensive research enquiry remains necessary in this area, particularly in terms of outcomes for clients, this is examined more closely in the chapter by Mary FitzGerald and Ysanne Chapman, Chapter 1.

This chapter however gives some clear messages about these students' experiences and offers what seem to be useful practical tips to support and motivate a novice reflector. There are also issues and concerns here for educationalists working with students and mentors who are developing reflective practice.

The perspectives presented appear to demonstrate to us that reflection has challenged the way that these practitioners think and feel about their practice (Burnard 1989). This in turn appears to have created practitioners who purport to be curious and open minded about their work rather than unquestioning and traditionally set in routine (Fay 1987). We would suggest that this has to be a positive thing for today's practitioners; in the words of the practitioner below,

'everyone has different experiences, there is no right or wrong, there is no perfect way to deal with one individual family. You will always learn something from it and even if you don't have a good experience it doesn't mean that you don't learn from it. I think that you have to be non-judgemental and perhaps reflection is the best way of dealing with palliative care and death and dying. How can you say that this is the perfect way (to practise) and every person should do it this way.'

Table 6.1   Practical tips

(1)	Use a reflective framework (e.g. Gibbs 1988) – stick it on your notice board above your desk where you study; refer to it as you work on your first jottings.
(2)	Get something down on paper as early as possible, not necessarily something academic or part of assessed work but something you can check out with your mentor in the first instance.
(3)	Keeping a reflective diary is helpful for some – write down what happened and why, what did I learn and what would I do next time?
(4)	Look back over your diary – use it to inform the academic work required of you.
(5)	Make sure you fix up an early meeting with your mentor – and keep it! Check your mentor knows what is expected of both of you.
(6)	Develop a repertoire of practice to draw on, store up experiences that you could use later in your reflective work, by making notes, jotting things down so that important experiences are not lost.
(7)	Get to know your mentor; use opportunities for reflective conversations.
(8)	If you can, get to know your tutor, make the most of any individual or group opportunities to get feedback.
(9)	Write down some reflection, then leave it – go away for a while (about two days) You may find it easier to be critical on your return.
(10)	If you are using a framework – refer to it and ensure all stages are covered in order to complete your analysis.
(11)	Go deep not wide in your analysis.
(12)	Live with lack of perfection – realise you won't always achieve the ideal, do what you can with some sense of direction.
(13)	Seek out colleagues who can and do support you.

References

Allen, D.G., Bowers, B. & Diekelmann, N. (1989) Writing to learn: A conceptualisation of thinking and writing in the nursing curriculum. *Journal of Nursing Education*, **28**, 6-11.

Basch, P. (1987) Focus group interviews; an under-utilised technique for improving theory and practice in health education. *Health Education Quarterly*, **14**, 411–47.

Boud, D., Keogh, R. & Walker, D. (1985) *Reflection: Turning Experience into Learning*, Kogan Page, London.

Burnard, P. (1989) Developing critical ability in nurse education. *Nurse Education Today*, **11** (2), 271–5.

Burrows, D. (1995) The nurse teacher's role in the promotion of reflective practice. *Nurse Education Today*, **15**, 346–50.

Carr, E.C.J. (1996) Reflecting on clinical practice: hectoring talk or reality? *Journal of Clinical Nursing*, **5**, 289–95.

Daloz, L.A. (1986) *Effective Teaching and Mentoring*, Jossey Bass Ltd, London.

Fay, B. (1987) *Critical Social Theory*, Polity Press, Cambridge.

French, P. & Cross, D. (1992) An interpersonal-epistemological curriculum model for nurse education. *Journal of Advanced Nursing*, **17**, 83–9.

Gibbs, G. (1988) *Learning by Doing: A guide to teaching and learning methods*, Further Education Unit, Oxford Polytechnic, Oxford.

Hargreaves, J. (1997) Using patients: exploring the ethical dimension of reflective practice in nurse education. *Journal of Advanced Nursing*, **25**, 223–8.

Heinrich, K.T. (1992) The intimate dialogue: journal writing by students. *Nurse Educator*, **17**, (6), Nov/Dec.

Holm, D. & Stephenson, S. (1994) Reflection – a student's perspective. In Palmer, A., Burns, S. & Bulman, C. (eds) *Reflective Practice in Nursing: The Growth of the Professional Practitioner*, Blackwell Science, Oxford, pp 53–62.

James, C.R. & Clarke, B.A. (1994) Reflective practice in nursing: issues and implications for nursing education. *Nurse Education Today*, **14**, 82–90.

Johns, C. (1995) The value of reflective practice for nursing. *Journal of Clinical Nursing*, **4**, 23–30.

McElroy, A. (1997) Developing the nurse teacher's role: the use of multiple focus groups to ensure grassroots involvement. *Nurse Education Today*, **17**, 145–9.

Mezirow, J. (1981) A critical theory of adult learning and education. *Adult Education*, **32** (1), 3–24.

Palmer, A., Burns, S. & Bulman, C. (eds) (1994) *Reflective Practice in Nursing: The Growth of the Professional Practitioner*, Blackwell Science, Oxford.

Paterson, B. (1995) Developing and maintaining reflection in clinical journals. *Nurse Education Today*, **15**, 211–20.

Schön, D. (1991) *The Reflective Practitioner*, second edn,. Jossey Bass, San Francisco.

Van Manen, M. (1977) Linking ways of knowing with ways of being practical. *Curriculum Inquiry*, **6** (3), 205–27.

Wellard, S.J. & Bethune, E. (1996) Reflective journal writing in nurse education: whose interests does it serve? *Journal of Advanced Nursing*, **24**, 1077–82.

Our thanks go to those listed below who were willing to take part in our focus group and enlightened us with their experiences of reflection.

Jane Bake, Lyn Back, Sally Harrison, Geraldine O'Meara, Gaye Hyle, Jackie Pateman, Catherine Wilson, Gillian Sykes, Rachel Pinder.

Chapter 7
The Experience of Becoming Reflective

Introduction

This is my story about becoming reflective and, although biased, I offer it in the hope that it will encourage and enthuse other practitioners to 'have a go'. When I first heard about reflection I thought that it was something completely irrelevant to me, partly because I did not understand what was being talked about, and partly because I thought that it was what I did in the car on the way home. This chapter explains what happened to make me change my mind and to begin experimenting with reflection.

The discussion is constructed from a number of themes from my reflective journals (Figure 7.1) that illustrate how my reflection developed over time and how it has contributed to the development of my practice and expertise. For example, reflection has helped me to transfer skills from my clinical practice to my education, research and management practice, thus enabling an integration of the various aspects of my role as a lecturer practitioner (LP). The discussion is illustrated by extracts from my reflective journals, in which all names have been changed.

'Better have a go'	Using reflection for different types of
Illuminating practice	practice
Analysing practice	Using reflection to transfer skills
Eliciting Knowledge	Helping other people to reflect
The personal cost of reflection	Critical friends
Change	Linking thinking and doing

Fig. 7.1   Themes arising from reflective journals 1991–1998.

Better have a go

When I first heard about reflection, it was discussed in such a hallowed way I thought that it was something mysterious – something to do with education and irrelevant to me. However, this discussion nagged at me and I began to try and understand what it was all about. With some relief I jumped at the idea that it was what I did in the car on the way home from work. Thus, like many nurses, I thought that it was something that I was already doing (Reid 1993).

My perception of reflection changed as a result of a lightly taken decision. I had been involved in planning a course that was going to encourage students to keep a reflective journal. A few weeks before the course began, I decided that I'd 'better have a go' before asking the students to do the same. However, completely unexpectedly, an early entry in my journal changed my understanding of reflection and made a powerful impact on me. This is what I wrote at the end of a shift on a hospice inpatient ward:

> 'Nursed a patient tired of fighting, feeling hopeless. I stayed with the patient but my heart emptied of anything that could protect me'. (18/9/91)

When I re-read this entry a month later, I was stunned how my feelings about caring for this person had been captured. I wondered 'how many times in the past had I felt like this and forgotten how I felt and why?' (22/9/91). This was a revelation to me. I realised for the first time that the habit of debriefing myself in the car, although helpful as a coping strategy, was causing me to forget the things I was doing in practice and I was losing the opportunity to learn from these experiences. This made such an impact on me that I wrote up the experience in more detail (Duke 1992). Although this account is superficial in terms of any analysis, it represents to me, in a very personal way, how written reflection can illuminate practice and the importance of writing and recording something (anything) about practice experiences.

Illuminating practice

Following this experience, I was determined to try and capture my clinical practice within my journal. However, I found the rigour and discipline of writing regularly difficult, and long periods of time elapsed between entries. In addition, although the entries record salient examples of palliative care practice, they are descriptive and this is due to a number of factors.

First, I did not find it easy to articulate my practice knowledge. When I first started to experiment with journal writing I had worked in palliative care settings for eight years. I was used to taking the short cuts in my assessment and decision making that Benner (1984) calls intuition. Intuitive practice is characterised by a conviction that what you are doing is the right and only course of action and the inability to describe to others (or to yourself) how you know this (Benner 1984). Later, I will describe my attempts at articulating intuitive knowledge, but for now it is important to recognise that the quality of my early reflective journal entries was influenced by both the certainty in practice that comes of being an expert and the difficulty of explaining how you know something. For example:

> 'M has been an inpatient for a long while ... She was a young person, in her late thirties and single. Her "fighting spirit" and determination to live is demonstrated by her comment: "if the body can make cancer then it can heal it". When we came on duty the night staff told us that M was restless and breathless and probably dying ... An alarm immediately went off in my head and I knew that M would probably die a difficult death.'

There is nothing in the reflection that directly follows this extract to illuminate why I felt that M would probably die a difficult death. In addition, the account describes how other people perceived the situation differently and the difficulty I had in convincing them that they were 'wrong' – in other words it illuminates my conviction that I was 'right' without any consideration that I might be 'wrong':

> '... the staff nurse came out of M's room looking very concerned and said that there wasn't enough written up to help her ... and that more sedation was needed. I challenged this and suggested that because M was frightened and fighting to live, this might not work, and that it may not be appropriate to make M unaware (to sedate her). ... I suggested that staying with M was as likely to help as drugs. Another staff nurse suggested that as M had always had people (friends and family) with her, staying with her now was unlikely to have the same effect as if this were a new thing to her. I suggested that the quality of the intervention would make a difference rather than the actual presence of someone. ... I just felt that whatever we did, M would die reluctantly because of her determination to live.' (28/4/92)

The second reason for the accounts being descriptive is that I did not see the need to analyse the incidents that I recorded. As an 'expert' I could recognise the issues that the accounts were illuminating. For example:

> 'Patient I cared for – young professor, condition deteriorating. At lunchtime I asked him if he would like something to eat. He thought about this (brain tumour so thinking now slow) and eventually said, "I feel very strongly about singing [few moments silence] but not eating" so I found an English music CD and put it on for him and then he went to sleep. Died a day later.' (20/2/03)

There is no analysis of this entry in my journal. Looking at it now, many things jump out from it that need expanding such as the ethics of my action, for example, in respect to offering music instead of food. Moreover, the entries are written in a way that forbids comment. They are presented as sacred representations of practice. They spoke to me about the nature of my practice and the power of nursing to influence the experience of people that I was caring for. Thus these early entries were akin to narratives and retold my experience (Richardson 1995).

The likeness between my reflective entries and narratives can be explained by what I was trying to achieve at the time. During this period I was trying to be credible to the practitioners that I was working with. I was trying to capture *evidence* of my practice knowledge in an attempt to justify my role. I therefore negated the possibility of using reflection to *expand* this knowledge. Some of the entries are quite short, such as the one that is depicted above. However, some are more detailed and try to elaborate the practice knowledge that I am trying to capture. For example, in the entry describing my experience of caring for M I wrote that she 'looked very frightened'. I went on to substantiate this opinion, to give evidence for it: 'her eyes were wide open and haunted, and she was breathing rapidly, working very hard to breathe. Her colour was grey'. Moreover, the whole account is designed to validate my initial assessment that M would die a difficult death. It goes on to describe the distress she experienced because she was dying and yet still 'fighting to live'.

The third reason for my accounts being descriptive is that my personal understanding of reflection was still emerging. About a year after commencing a journal, I reviewed the clinical practice entries and formulated the framework that I was using as that depicted in Figure 7.2. Note that I depicted reflection as something separate although related to

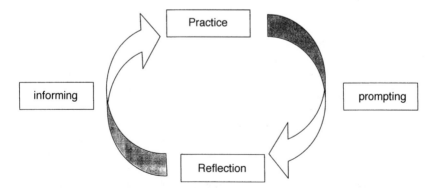

Fig. 7.2 Illustrating early model of reflection used in reflective journal.

practice despite knowing about Schön's (1983) concept of reflection-in-action. My diary entries typically included a description of an incident, my feelings about it, and some evaluation as to what went well and not so well.

Analysing practice

The descriptive nature of my reflection changed little by little as I began to consider underpinning meanings to the incidents I reflected upon. I do not remember this development as a conscious one but rather as an evolutionary one that was possible because of the increasing number of entries in my journal. When I read back over these accounts, I began to identify common issues and concepts within them. I then began proactively to explore these concepts using relevant research and theory and then used the outcome of this exploration to inform my clinical practice.

This was a very exciting period because I was actively engaged in researching my practice in the way that Schön (1983) describes and I was directing my own learning about practice and the adequacy of theory and research to explain it. Writing in my journal became less of a chore. I typified Mezirow's (1991) description of a student propelled by and absorbed in what I was doing. As a result, I became more willing to pull the accounts apart. I made the time and had the energy to learn what questions to ask of my accounts and this in turn increased my reflection in clinical practice. Thus, I finally integrated reflection-on-action with reflection-in-action (Schön 1983) and the reflective process I followed became active and dynamic (Figure 7.3).

Depicting this interconnection between practice and theoretical exploration is difficult to illustrate because it was a very dynamic process. Looking at my journals, what seems to have happened is that a theme emerged through a number of entries, I then explored it theoretically and in practice. Thus, no one theme is linked with any particular practice incident. In fact, many themes arise from all of the examples in my journal at this time. The following synopsis draws out how one concept, empowerment, was explored and how it impacted on my practice.

Three practice incidents record empowerment as a theme prior to it being explored theoretically. The three incidents take place over an eight-month period. The first relates to the advice that I gave to another nurse that enabled her to discuss a patient's diagnosis and prognosis with her. The second describes how I addressed a patient's fear of morphine, using information so that he could make informed choices

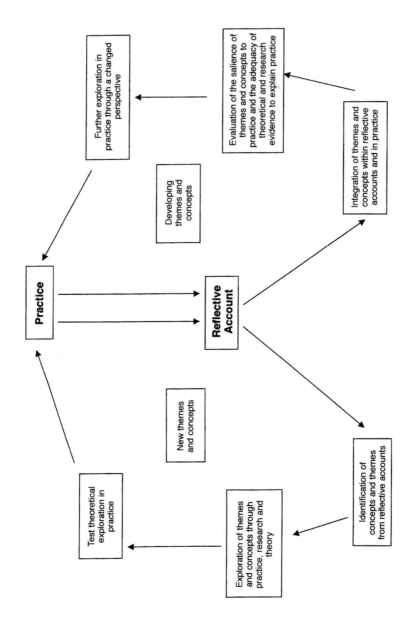

Fig. 7.3 Reflection as an active process.

about using this drug for pain relief. The third describes how I felt about a patient who responded to his diagnosis in a very passive and dependent way and how I tried to give him choices about his care so that he could increase his participation.

These incidents prompted an exploration of empowerment using a range of research and literature and experimentation in my practice to try and increase the amount of interaction that I had with colleagues, patients and family members, particularly in respect to understanding what was happening. For example, when nursing a young person with a rapidly progressive pneumonia, I wrote

> 'I worked hard at keeping the patient, the family and the SHO up to date with A's condition. I hoped that this would help the family be prepared for bad news. I spent time explaining what was happening, what I was doing and why and tried to give them the information they needed to make decisions about treatment'. (29/3/93)

Eliciting knowledge

As a result of this interactive use of reflection, my journal entries became more detailed. I commenced a period in my reflection where I tried very hard to be explicit about practice in the way described by Benner (1984) and within critical incident technique (Flanagan 1954). I constructed a summary of theories about knowledge as a framework to analyse the reflective accounts (Fig. 7.4) and was particularly interested in the artistic knowledge elicited by this process.

Two types of entries are typical of this effort. The first documents or captures intuitive insights into practice: 'introduced myself and very clearly saw a person with terminal agitation, the term just jumped into my mind' (20/4/94). The second tries to draw out the knowledge embedded in practice, and is illustrated below. The account centres on Sally, a 47 year old woman with two children and living apart from her husband. She had a close and supportive relationship with her sister Hazel. On the morning I met her I had been asked to give her a wash by the ward co-ordinator. Sally was distressed because her sister was leaving. As I spent time with her, I realised that she was confused and frightened about what was happening. Using what she was able to tell me and the cues from her behaviour and the environment I worked out that she was hypercalcaemic and being treated with a bisphosphonate. I also guessed that she was experiencing side effects from metaclopromide, a drug that had been given to manage nausea and vomiting resulting from the hypercalcaemia.

	Summary
Theoretical knowledge	Empirics: 'the process wherein evidence is rooted in objective reality and gathered through human senses is used as the basis of gathering knowledge' – objective, factual, generalisable and publicly verifiable (Carper 1978). Propositional knowledge or textbook knowledge – knowing that rather than knowing how (Heron 1981). You *know* something if you fulfil the certain conditions: that you *know* that what they say is true; that you are sure of it; that you have a right to be sure (Ayer 1956).
Artistic knowledge	Esthetic, the art of nursing, to do with empathy, understanding and perceiving and involves technical skills and an understanding what is significant in an individual's behaviour (Carper 1978). Practical knowledge (Benner 1984), linked with intuitive knowledge as a sign of an expert. Benner argues that practical problems require engagement, attentiveness and conceptual reasoning and outlines 6 areas of practical knowledge: graded qualitative distinction; common meanings; assumption (certain courses of events that are expected); (predisposition to act in certain ways); paradigm cases and personal knowledge (approach a situation using past experience); maxims (Polyani (1969) calls these rules of art); unplanned practices. Ayer (1956) suggests that intuition is something known without knowing why it is known i.e. there is no evidence for this knowing and trying to understand the basis of this knowing logically, reduces it. The capacity to receive sensations or impressions and that intuition is apprehensions and awareness of objects of experience – communicated through beauty and the skill and requires imagination and understanding (Kant, cited in Speake, 1979). Knowing how rather than knowing that (Heron 1981).
Personal knowledge	Personal knowledge is to do with the way in which individual nurses view themselves and the client – therapeutic use of self and the nature of the interpersonal process being subjective, concrete, existential, whole and integral (Carper 1978). Experiential knowledge – that gained by personal experience (Heron 1981).
Ethical knowledge	'the understanding of different positions about what is good, right and wrong' (Carper 1978). The beliefs and values underpinning practice (Heron 1981).

Fig. 7.4 Framework for analysing knowledge embedded in reflective entries.

Excerpt	Type of knowledge
'[Sally's] sister is saying goodbye. I sit and just listen and try and feel what is going on. To do this I focus on Sally and her sister and still myself – try and empty myself and make room for Sally. Sally is fidgety, quick movements, sweaty, short phrases/words, and slurred, slightly muddled order. Mouth sticky. 'What are you going to do?' she asks me. I tell her [that I have been asked] to help her have a wash. 'A quick one'. I . . . give her a small wash and make her comfortable . . . spend time with her. This goes OK and afterwards she tells me that she doesn't know what is wrong with her. I reflect this phrase back to her and she says no one has told her anything. I say I think that she has had a drip because her blood chemistry is wrong. She is anxious because it hasn't helped yet. I say that it is unlikely to help so quickly. Sally says that she is feeling very ill, sick, aches in her back and sides and is very frightened, scared. There is no room to explore this very far . . . [or] ask her if she needs more information. The best I can do is to listen and meet her gaze and hold her hand – with this we make contact and she is more visibly relaxed.' (21/5/93)	Personal knowledge – how to encounter another person on a personal level, how to make contact, how to make sense of a situation. Artistic knowledge – assessment of Sally's condition and knowledge of salient issues. I wrote later that I concentrated on washing Sally 'fluently' so that her confidence in me would increase and so that her anxiety would decrease. I was also balancing the theoretical or empirical risks of pressure damage with her need for comfort (ethical knowledge). The care that I gave her seemed to have the effect of enabling her to talk to me about her concerns and gave me an opportunity to understand how I might be of help to her, how I might support her. Personal knowledge – the 'physical' care enables me to use myself in a way that enabled Sally to explore her fears. I tried to give her information that would help her to understand the situation more fully within the limits of her fear and anxiety. Empirical knowledge – knowledge of hypercalcaemia and its physiological effects and likely treatment, knowledge of side effects of metaclopromide.

This entry in my journal also marks the beginning of contextualising my practice experience by examining the milieu and culture in which it took place and thus I began to address socio-political knowledge (Heath 1998). I broadened my account to include what else was happening in the ward environment and influencing the care given. For example, in the above example, I wrote that my ability to give care to Sally was influenced by the shift co-ordinator

'concentrating on and encouraging us to focus on physical care for the people we are caring for, focusing on getting the work done rather than being with people (can work with people ever be done?!).'

Contextualising practice experience resulted in two significant shifts in my reflection. The first was a move from analysing the knowledge embedded in practice towards noticing discrepancies between what was being practised and the professed values and principles of palliative care

– the difference between what Argyris & Schön (1974) describe as the-ories-in-action and espoused theories. The second was a move from reflection resulting in changes in beliefs, attitudes and emotional reac-tions, to reflection resulting in a transformed understanding of the assumptions underpinning practice (Mezirow 1991). Thus, under-standing some of the cultural issues underpinning practice had, as Goodman (1984) suggests, led me to a deeper and very different level of reflection.

It is difficult to analyse how these shifts occurred. From my journal I know that it was not a planned change. My best guess is that the reflection I had engaged in thus far had enabled me to validate my knowledge and that this gave me confidence in practice that freed me to observe and to think about what was happening around me. This may be akin to what Munhall (1993) calls 'unknowing', where a practitioner moves away from expert practice that has resulted in closure, that is, confidence in one's own interpretation, to an open awareness of prac-tice. Whatever the explanation, I am fairly certain that it was a direct *repercussion* of previous reflective endeavours rather than simply a *sequential* progression in the acquisition of reflective skills. This shift led to a profound experience in the use of reflection that had a personal cost.

The personal cost of reflection

Recognising a discrepancy between what was being collectively pro-fessed and what was being practised was a personal watershed. It called into question all the assumptions that I had made about my clinical and teaching practice and led to a complete re-visioning of my practice. Mezirow (1991, p. 67) describes this process as perspective transfor-mation:

> 'the process of becoming critically aware of how and why our assumptions have come to constrain the way we perceive, understand and feel about our world; changing these structures of habitual expectation to make possible a more inclusive discriminating and integrative perspective; and finally, making choices or otherwise acting on this new understanding'.

My experience of this transformative process began by feeling con-fused by the incongruencies I was noticing. It was very difficult to accept the alternative perspective that my reflection was suggesting. I tried to prove that it was wrong, to put my insights aside – to repress them, but they kept nagging at me. I became very angry that not everyone was trying to put the ideologies of hospice care into practice as I was trying to do. I was angry with myself for blaming the difficulties that I had experienced as a lecturer practitioner on deficiencies in my knowledge and skills, whereas I could now see other explanations. I was also very sad and disappointed and mourned the loss of my innocent vision of palliative care. This was a difficult and exhausting time. For some months my journal is full of comments such as '...the end of a long week in which frustration and tiredness have been welling up', 'feeling very tired and weary', 'exhausted, physically and emotionally'.

There are also indications in my journal entries that it was a time when I really got to grips with many practice issues in a way I had not done before. I had a varying degree of success in this, not least because I was still angry and therefore not always tactful or very skilful in how I was raising this challenge. In addition, the transformation in my understanding of practice had made me different and I was therefore doing things that colleagues would not have expected of me. In some respects I was a traitor. I had deserted the collective view and was attacking the ideology held by many of my colleagues. I consequently encountered and experienced reactions that might be expected in this situation but which nevertheless felt very personal and painful. I had effectively committed what Brookfield (1993, p. 201) so eloquently describes as cultural suicide:

> 'the process by which ... in taking a critical stance toward conventional assumptions and procedures, (practitioners) face the prospect of finding themselves excluded from the culture that has defined and sustained them up to that point in their lives'

Change

Like the nurses in Brookfield's paper, I felt isolated and it took a long while for this feeling to change. I needed this time to work with and to understand this experience. This work was all encompassing and involved me as a person as well as a nurse. For example, I mentioned that I had believed that the difficulty that I had experienced in implementing the role of the lecturer practitioner in the unit was due to my lack of knowledge and skills. Although this probably had a measure of truth within it, I also became aware that this was a position I had been encouraged to believe by my past educational experience. I began to question this and my reflection became very reflexive (the self turned back on itself). Over a period of time I dealt with some ghosts from my childhood such as re-evaluating the beliefs engraved by schooling that resulted in my belief that I am not 'academic'. As a result, I learnt that I have dyslexic tendencies and I found deep scars within me relating to my feelings about being oppressed because of this. (I am still working on the negative feelings evoked by the word 'academic' but at least I can now recognise where they come from).

Alongside this work, I examined a number of theoretical concepts that made sense of the issues I was examining and the process involved. For example I was drawn to theory and research on oppression and found Rather's (1994) analysis of Freire's (1972) work particularly helpful in understanding how oppression results in powerlessness and inferiority through internalising the beliefs of the oppressor. So, although this was a very personal time in my reflection, I continued to use theory and research to help me make sense of my experiences.

Using reflection for different types of practice

Throughout my journals there is a relationship between the quality of my reflection and the expertise that I had developed in the practice on which I was reflecting. In addition, there seems to be a relationship between the rate of development in the particular practice and my increasing competence in the process of reflection. For example an early entry about teaching practice is more akin to a note or jotting:

> 'Today started teaching module x . . . Morning went well. Group very full of life. Great. Felt like I was throwing paper all over the place all the time. Well received though. Physiology test has stunned them. Good idea for next week – get into groups first thing to recap things learnt since this week/or what they remember about this week. Think I'll try it. Also – get sandwiches at coffee time! I'm relieved it went well – difficult to tell how well as so jammed pack and I don't know everyone very well yet'. (4/10/91)

I suspect that the quality of this reflection is partly to do with my limited knowledge and partly because of my lack of understanding about reflection at the time that it was written. I was unable to analyse my teaching practice because I was an inexperienced educational practitioner and unable to use reflection to help me to identify a focus to explore relevant educational theory and research because I was still learning how to reflect. However, as I become more accomplished in reflection, the quality of these entries change. For example, they begin to integrate description, analysis, theoretical exploration and how I responded and felt about my teaching experiences. Although the accounts do not demonstrate any intuitive insights, they do try and highlight the skills and knowledge underpinning the practice:

Student finding reflection threatening ... [she had written] that she felt angry that her tutors were [devaluing] her previous experience. My response initially on reading this was very defensive (protecting me because it made me feel inadequate and rekindled my feelings of being inexperienced). But then I was able to <u>honestly</u> accept what she was saying – I couldn't take responsibility for her past and her feelings or response to the course. I would be more help to her to be honest and accept her views and to take seriously my responsibility to her – which is to support, understand and value her as a person and as a student'. (11/5/92)

This piece of reflection then progressed to look at the influence of communication skills on interactions with students and some theory around self-directed learning. It also explored the moral responsibility involved in helping students look at issues related to death and dying:

'I have also began to understand the importance of supporting students and yet letting them experience the pain involved with being self-directed learners and with caring for the dying. I cannot take this on for them but I can support them while they experience it. More importantly, I realised last term that in order to learn from the experience and grow from it, students need to be open to the experience and reflect on it. I shouldn't try and protect them from it, or worry about their experience. I must understand that it is their experience and understand my role within this'.

Using reflection to transfer skills across different kinds of practice

Becoming more competent in the process of reflection also enabled me to identify similarities between different aspects of my practice. At first this recognition was unintentional. For example, in the entry above I wrote 'I became aware of using supportive and communication skills very similar to those that I use with patients and their families'. However, over time I began to notice similarities in both the skills that I used and in the way in which I expressed my practice (Figure 7.5). I began to use reflection to analyse these similarities, in order to transfer skills intentionally across different types of practice, in the way demonstrated in Figure 7.6. This intentional integration of skills across the different kinds of practice that I am engaged in has enabled me to expand my expertise in all facets of my role.

Clinical practice	Management practice
I tried to <u>feel</u> what E was saying to me ... I quietened myself ... I strained every sense to capture what I was being told' (9/91)	'... in meetings I listen carefully ready to add clarification and [ask] questions as needed ... This often means that all my attention is on what is being said rather than what is meant and there is little concentration left to me to <u>feel</u> the group ... I need to do something about this. I also need to develop enough confidence in my teaching that I can respond to what I feel in the group rather than worry that I might be wrong. I must start to test and trust my perceptions' (21/1/93)

Fig. 7.5   Comparison of reflective analysis between different types of practice.

Helping other people to reflect

As I have become more experienced in using reflection I have become more active in helping other people reflect. At first, this was limited to helping students with their reflective accounts by engaging in written dialogue. However, my reflection on practice has enabled me to know what sort of questions to ask other people about their reflection. For example, I asked a colleague reflecting on presence (something that I have spent a great deal of time reflecting upon):

'how do you know when you are able to be with people in this way? Can you say more about the quietness of your presence? How do you quieten yourself? How do you "be"? How does this differ from when you "do"? Does the ability to "be" depend on the other person's ability to receive someone else's being?' (17/1/98)

I have also found that letting other people see my reflection is a powerful way to illustrate what it is. This is particularly so when the reflection is about practice that they have also been engaged in. For instance, when collecting data for a study on the role of community Macmillan nurses (Duke *et al.* 1998), I wrote my observations of their practice in a field work diary and asked the nurses to comment on my observations and to try and answer the questions I was raising. Reading these observations made a powerful impact on one of the nurses involved, she described them as 'amazing', and they had helped her to value her practice and to ask questions of it.

On other occasions I have used this strategy intentionally with nurses

Practice example	Management example
'... Bert, 71, married, retired publican, Ca lung, bony secondaries, admitted five days ago with: 1. Confusion, disorientation time and place. 2. Pain and immobility – back and shoulders. Bert still very confused, most of conversation to this point had not made sense [and yet the following stood out]: Bert: "You don't know what to think of life, it's hard to know how to look at life, look at the good points and the bad points." SD [tentatively]: "I guess it's a mixture of both." Bert: "You're so right." Later (an hour or so): Bert: "Wouldn't it be wonderful if I was splashed across the newspapers having been cured?" SD: "Yes that would be lovely wouldn't it? Does this relate to what you were telling me earlier about life being good and bad, what to think of it?" Bert: "Yes it does" SD: "How realistic do you think cure is Bert?" Bert: "I know it isn't, I was just wishing." (27/4/93)	Context is a clinical management meeting. Some discussion about my working the weekend and whether this is appropriate use of my time and whether it would be possible for me to give more warning about this. I reply [to each point] ... I can't understand all this discussion about my working the weekend, I had given plenty of notice and the ward had been busy and I was able to constructively contribute to the care. (29/4/93)

Issues:

Q: Why had I not recognised any cues within the meeting that would have helped me to address the issues that were trying to be raised?

A: I was replying to what was being said but not listening to what was not being said, as I had been able to in the clinical practice example.

Plan: To try and listen to what is not being said in meetings and use the literature to explore cues and perception further. (3/5/93)

Fig. 7.6 Transferring skills across practice.

who want to examine an aspect of their practice. For example, the questions quoted above about presence are taken from swapped reflective accounts with a staff nurse following negotiated observation of her practice (requested by her). I was stunned by the similarity in our reflection and by this nurse's very profound depth of thinking and sensitivity to the practice we had been engaged in. I have found that written reflection has the potential to elicit a depth of analysis that is hard to capture verbally. Thus sharing written accounts requires sensitivity to their potential power and the possibilities that they can 'stun' someone into silence (block learning) as well as the potential to stimulate participative dialogue.

Critical friends

Although reflective journals have been important vehicles for developing my reflective skills – I have used them to 'write [myself] into understanding' (Heinrich 1992, p. 17). I have needed support and critical dialogue from colleagues to sustain this activity. Sometimes colleagues have acted as a sounding board for my ideas and thoughts, sometimes they have given me an 'expert' view of an area of knowledge new to me, and sometimes they have stimulated a thought that I have then gone on to explore.

In addition to this informal support and dialogue, my reflection has occasionally been supported by supervision. I use supervision as a focus for testing out and planning action in response to my reflection. My current supervisor recently commented that supervision appeared to be irrelevant other than it providing a date by which to think something through and an opportunity to engage in what he and others call reflection-before-action (Greenwood 1993). However, this negates the thinking that goes on after the meeting and the nature of the debate raised. This debate is akin to what Carr & Kemmis (1986) call dialectical, which is about searching out contradictions and moving beyond them. For example, my supervisor recently challenged me to consider the incongruency between what I am trying to achieve (a collegial, participative approach to management) and my decision on how to act in response to a particular incident (head on, confrontational, authoritative). This challenge enabled me to consider other ways of acting; in this particular instance I acted by doing nothing. In addition, supervision helps me to explore how I 'be' when I act. For example, we recently explored my assessment of my actions in a classroom and how I was able to help people learn rather than just teach them:

> 'the students were saying how difficult it was to learn about the physiology of pain and instead of going over the content again as I have done in the past I explained why this might be and we discussed why learning is hard'. (Nov 1998)

Linking thinking and doing

Thus, the intrinsic purpose of supervision is action that is based on careful thought and sensitive being; something done that will positively change practice intentionally, mindful of my own and other's integrity. Supervision helps me to act wisely and patiently (although this is *very* frustrating at times). It weaves my practice and reflection together to create what Mezirow (1991) calls reflective action, a dynamic dialectic (see above) between thought and action. Reflective action both recreates my understanding of a situation and transforms the situation (Figure 7.7).

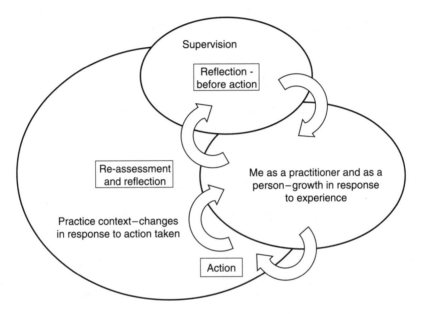

Fig. 7.7   Dynamic relationship between thinking and doing.

The relationship between thinking and doing has been described as praxis (Carr & Kemmis 1986) and practical wisdom (Lauder 1994), concepts that I am trying to gain a clearer understanding of in order to progress further with my understanding of reflection. It is here that my story ends. Although I am unsure of what will happen next, I am certain that it is not the end of my experience of becoming reflective because reflection has become part of me. It is about who I am as a person, and if I have an intention to continue to grow as a person reflection will always be part of my life. I have more sense of the need to 'be' (to live reflection), rather than to 'do' it (to write reflection as a separate activity). I have begun to understand that it is a very powerful thing to be able to demonstrate the quintessential nature of reflection through living it.

Conclusion

In this chapter I have tried to translate my experience of becoming reflective through an analysis of my reflective journals. As noted at the beginning, there are problems with this endeavour; it is biased because it is about my experience. However, I have tried to recreate this experience as honestly as possible, letting it speak for itself, rather than drawing it into an analysis based on available comment and research. Perhaps this is for others to do as they assess the helpfulness, or not, of what I have written. Nevertheless, I hope that the essential message of this experience is clear; you can not comment on reflection unless you have 'had a go' because until then you will never know what reflection is. Although reflection takes time to develop and can have personal costs, it has the power to enlighten, empower and emancipate (Fay 1987). It can't be 'done' or reduced to mechanistic techniques (Greenwood 1998, Richardson 1995). Reflection needs to be lived and experienced.

References and further reading

Argyris, C. & Schön, D. (1974) *Theory in Practice: Increasing Professional Effectiveness*, Addison Wesley, Massachusetts.

Ayer, A.J. (1956) *The Problem of Knowledge*, Penguin, London.

Benner, P. (1984) *From Novice to Expert*, Addison Wesley, Massachusetts.

Brookfield, S. (1993) On impostorship, cultural suicide and other danger: How nurses learn critical thinking. *The Journal of Continuing Education in Nursing*, **24** (5), 197–205.

Carper, B.A. (1978) Fundamental patterns of knowing in nursing, *Advances in Nursing Science*, **1** (1), 13–23.

Carr, W. & Kemmis, S. (1986) *Becoming Critical*, The Falmer Press, London.

Duke, S. (1992) Space to speak. *Nursing Times*, **88** (23), 49.

Duke, S., Prowse, S., Fancott, J. & Dancer, J. (1998) *Palliative care need assessment of Central and West Oxfordshire*, Report available from Sir Michael Sobell House, Oxford.

Fay, B. (1987) *Critical Social Science*, Polity Press, Cambridge.

Flanagan, J.C. (1954) The critical incident technique. *Psychological Bulletin*, **51** (4), 327–58.

Freire, P. (1972) *Pedagogy of the Oppressed*, Penguin, London.

Goodman, J. (1984) Reflection and teacher education: a case study and theoretical analysis. *Interchange*, **15** (3), 9–25.

Greenwood, J. (1993) Reflective practice: a critique of the work of Argyris and Schön. *Journal of Advanced Nursing*, **19**, 1183–7.

Greenwood, J. (1998) The role of reflection in single and double loop learning. *Journal of Advanced Nursing*, **27**, 1048–53.

Heath, H. (1998) Reflection and patterns of knowing. *Journal of Advanced Nursing*, **27**, 1054–59.

Heinrich, K.T. (1992) The intimate dialogue: Journal writing by students. *Nurse Educator*, **17** (6), 17–21.

Heron, J. (1981) Philosophical basis for a new paradigm. Chapter 2 in Reason, P. & Rowan, A. (eds) *Human Inquiry: A Sourcebook for a New Paradigm Research*, John Wiley, London.

Lauder, W. (1994) Beyond reflection: practical wisdom and the practical syllogism. *Nurse Education Today*, **14**, 91–8.

Mezirow, J. (1991) How critical reflection triggers transformative learning. Chapter 1 in Mezirow, J. (ed) *Fostering Critical Reflection in Adulthood*, Jossey-Bass, San Francisco, pp. 1–20.

Munhall, P. (1993) 'Unknowing': towards another pattern of knowing in nursing. *Nursing Outlook*, **41** (3), 125–8.

Polyani, M. (1969) *Knowing and Being*, University of Chicago Press, Chicago.

Rather, M.L. (1994) Schooling for oppression: A hermeneutical analysis of the lived experience of the returning RN student. *Journal of Nursing Education*, **33** (6), 263–71.

Reid, B. (1993) But we're doing it already! Exploring a response to the concept of reflective practice in order to improve its facilitation. *Nurse Education Today*, **13**, 305–9.

Richardson, R. (1995) Humpty Dumpty: reflection and reflective practice. *Journal of Advanced Nursing*, **21**, 1044–50.

Schön, D. (1983) *The Reflective Practitioner*, Temple Smith, London.

Speake, J. (1979) (ed) *A Dictionary of Philosophy*, Pan, London.

Chapter 8
The Legacy of Reflective Practice

'My experience of reflection is continuous. It is an ingrained part of the nursing care I ... offer children and their families and it dictates my actions. It has formed the backbone of my practice aiding my professional and personal progression in ... nursing' (Wooton 1997, p. 6).

Introduction

This chapter explores the extent to which reflective practice introduced to student nurses during their training continues to have a legacy after they become qualified nurses. First the perceived advantages of including reflection within the curriculum are outlined. This is followed by a review of the literature relating to this area. Finally the findings of a study into the experiences of newly qualified children's nurses are discussed, particularly those pertaining to the influence of reflection on these qualified nurses.

Why teach reflective skills?

There is a school of thought that nurse education is a system of indoctrination or socialisation and that the educational programme which the students undertake plays a significant role in this process (Lamond 1974 Simpson 1979, Holloway & Penson 1987, Bassett 1993). Arguably, when individuals first embark on their nursing career they have few insights into their role. They gain the knowledge and skills required for practice and assimilate the norms, values and attitudes of those around them during their academic work and their practice experience. In these ways they become increasingly aware of the expectations of others and develop a tendency to emulate the behaviour expected by the profession. This is all instrumental in helping to shape their future practice and may leave them with the particular attributes and characteristics of life long learning and an overall professional identity (Lowe & Kerr 1998).

It has been suggested by Dewey (1933) that this learning can take place in two ways; either by trial and error or by engaging in reflective activity. Prior to 1986, traditional nurse training was based upon an apprenticeship system and tended to support the former approach. However, perhaps as a result of the impetus to equip practitioners with critical and analytical skills, learning by reflection seems to have gathered momentum during the last decade and the new educational pathways, post 1986 (i.e. Project 2000 Diploma in Higher Education – DipHe – and degrees), have emphasised the purposeful nature and value of the latter (James & Clarke 1994, Hallett 1997a). This is described by Entwhistle & Ramsden (1983) as a combination of personal learning and formal learning which results in 'deep learning'.

Initially this change in emphasis seems to have emanated from a desire by educators and service managers to address some of the deficits of previous training. The belief is that reflection has several lasting benefits. Pierson (1998) anticipated that this approach to thinking about practice leaves a legacy with the nurses after they have qualified:

(1)   It may reduce the reality shock experienced by newly qualified staff nurses, popularised by Kramer (1968, 1974, 1985), by offering them a tool to be used to make sense of their world of practice. It is envisaged that if the practitioners are so equipped with the ability to analyse complex situations this may in turn reduce their stress and enhance their coping strategies in the early stages of their careers (Dearmun 1998).

(2)   It is claimed that reflection can be used to integrate theory and practice and advance learning from experience (Haddock & Bassett 1997). This stimulates ideas for research and has perceived benefits for clients, although this is yet to be verified.

(3)   Reflection may increase self awareness and insight into behaviour and responses in relation to particular situations; thus enabling practitioners to analyse their relationships with others in the social setting. In this way it can be used as a strategy for self management and self improvement.

(4)   This approach to learning has utility for the service agenda surrounding quality of care and clinical governance (Johns 1994, Kohner 1994, NHSME 1998) because many of the skills generated through reflection mirror those required to maximise the value of clinical supervision.

(5)   Given the above agenda, service managers may favour practitioners who have a propensity to analyse their practice critically. Through this process it is probable that such personnel will find new, imaginative ways of working and will be able to respond to

situations in the ever changing practice arena. (See Bev Gillings' chapter, Chapter 5, on clinical supervision and reflection.)

In these ways it can be seen that reflection could be used extensively by educators as a means of integrating theory and practice and encouraging students to learn from their experience and it could also have a wider appeal beyond the initial training period. The literature is replete with academic and practice discussion papers on reflection (for example, Jarvis 1992, Atkins & Murphy 1993, Pierson 1998) and nearly all pre-registration nursing programmes at DipHE and degree level, validated by the English National Board, now have reflection as a key theme within the curriculum. A definitive definition remains elusive and it is common for a course philosophy to be underpinned by several theories of reflection (for example, Dewey 1938, Argryis & Schön 1974, Mezirow 1981; Schön 1983, 1987, Gibbs 1988, Boud *et al.* 1985, Palmer *et al.* 1994). These in turn tend to inform the student's perceptions of reflection during their course. The hallmarks of these theories include an analysis of all aspects of practice situations in order to identify what has been learnt and an appraisal of the knowledge and skills used and those required to address future situations more effectively with new insights. Various methods are introduced to educate student nurses to be able to reflect systematically on their practice. These include, among others, the analysis of critical incidents in reflective essays and the use of diaries (Richardson *et al.* 1995). (See Chapter 3 on assessment and evaluation for further examples.)

Overall there seems to have been assumptions, and in some cases a conviction that the process of reflection can be taught (Schön 1987, Van Manen 1991), or at least fostered in part, by the educational programme that nurses have undertaken. This has led to some attempts to evaluate the extent to which reflection informs an individual's practice during his or her training. For example, the reflective learning contract approach and the grading of students' reflective accounts were developed in Oxford, to assess clinical practice (Burns 1992, Dearmun 1997a, Wooton 1997, Harding 1998).

What influences the use of reflection after a nurse qualifies?

Students may respond differently to the use of reflection and demonstrate different levels of reflective abilities and skills. Undoubtedly for some the tendency to reflect may be an inherent characteristic which they already possess and this is merely stirred by the introduction of this methodical approach to learning. For others it is something that is quite novel and they accept it enthusiastically and have little difficulty incorporating it into their practice. Unfortunately there will be a number of students who do not feel comfortable with reflection and never really grasp this approach. Consequently they may feel that they are coerced into thinking in this way in order to fulfil the requirements of the course and may be more likely to reject it as soon as they qualify.

It could be argued that the lasting benefits of reflection and becoming and being a life long reflective proactive practitioner may only be realised if nurses internalise the process and continue to work in a reflective manner after completion of their initial educational programme. So apart from their personal characteristics what else influences this?

There have been relatively few published empirical studies that have examined the lasting influence of reflection. Powell (1989) observed nurse–patient interaction and used interviews to explore the extent to which practitioners continued to use reflection when they qualified. Two particularly relevant findings emerged. First there were indications that DipHE nurses seemed to be dominated by rules and laws and it was speculated that nurses educated to degree level would be more reflective and analytical. Second, a rigid work culture that was hierarchical, prescriptive of practice and intolerant of change tended to reinforce the nurses' adherence to a technical–rationality model of care (Schön 1983). It is reasonable to assume therefore that this in turn may inhibit reflection. For example, as a result of engaging in the reflective process a nurse may perceive that there is a need to re-examine and alter his or her own practice or persuade others to change their ways of working. The organisational structures may or may not give nurses the autonomy to do this. Dearmun (1997b) traced the impact of the milieu in which individuals find themselves working after qualifying and found it to be influential in terms of enhancing or inhibiting a nurse's tendency to be overtly reflective. So it seems that the mode and level of education a nurse receives could be a factor in promoting his or her reflective abilities but the organisational culture can also play a significant part.

McCaughterty (1991) used an experimental design to evaluate the introduction of reflection into the curriculum as a method of integrating theory and practice. The teaching model focused on the nurses' ability to provide a theoretical rationale for the care they had given but did not encourage them to challenge the theory or acknowledge their feelings about situations. Despite the limitations of the study, there were indications that when nurses were given a chance to discuss their experiences they displayed a depth of understanding and empathy for the clients they were nursing and this may be a precursor to reflection.

It has been suggested by Rolfe (1997) that in order to foster reflection at least three factors have to be present:

- a particular state of mind
- an acute awareness of the clinical situation
- and a relationship with an individual client.

A fourth dimension may be the opportunity to share reflections with another person; a feature identified by Schön (1987) and supported by Hallett *et al.* (1996). It was found that being coached by supervisors in the skills of reflection provided the opportunity for practitioners to make sense of their experiences. It has also been found that the disposition to reflect has a chronological dimension and is associated with the length of time spent in practice (Dearmun 1997b). There is a plausible explanation for this. The early experiences of practice are disorientating and confusing because initially practitioners do not fully understand what they are doing. Consequently they spend considerable time mastering the necessary practical techniques and skills in order to feel comfortable in the practice environment and be accepted by the team. Without the practice experience they find it is difficult to apply the theories they have learnt in the classroom. With more time in practice their confidence grows and they begin to see the relevance of what they have been taught. At about six months there is a resurgence in their reflection. This notion of increased time spent in practice as being pivotal to learning, and possibly reflection, has been central to the theses in previous studies (Benner 1984, Benner *et al.* 1996, MacLeod 1996).

Does reflection have a legacy?

Until recently, there have been no published studies taking a longitudinal approach to exploring this phenomenon after initial pre-registration education. The main purpose of this chapter is to share the findings of a study that considered the legacy of reflective practice.

In 1997 a research study was undertaken into the perceptions of newly qualified children's nurses (Dearmun 1997b). The subsidiary aims of this study were to consider the extent to which a BA (Hons) Paediatric Nursing course, which was grounded on the notion of reflection, continued to influence nurses when they graduated, and to explore the extent to which nurses continued to use reflection as a tool for the systematic analysis of their practice and to learn from their experience.

All nurses who graduated from the BA (Hons) Children's Nursing course were interviewed about their experiences of being staff nurses.

The study was based within the naturalistic paradigm because the intention was to explore the *emic* view or to gain the nurses' perspectives of their experiences during the first year after qualifying. The nurses' views were ascertained in two ways: through interactive interviews conducted on four occasions during the year and the use of pictorial narratives to trace the progression in their thoughts and feelings over the year. By using this longitudinal design it was possible to capture the changes in the nurses' perceptions as they evolved over a period of time. All the interviews were tape recorded and transcribed verbatim. Data was then analysed using some of the tenets of grounded theory and constant comparative analysis (Glaser & Strauss 1967). The data was coded and themes were identified.

During the interviews the nurses volunteered information about the myriad of influences on their practice. For the most part they talked spontaneously about reflective practice, giving examples of situations in which they had used reflection. They expressed many sentiments that indicated that this concept continued to have some relevance for them during the year after they qualified.

The nurses' feelings about reflection

It was clear that the nurses had positive and negative feelings about reflection. At first some of them had mixed feelings about it but at the point at which they qualified most of them gave indications that they valued having developed an ability to analyse their practice.

Those that expressed a negative view were aware of the adverse effects reflection could have. One participant suggested that during the course they felt they had been forced to analyse thoughts, feelings and actions and this had been detrimental, painful and had undermined their confidence.

> 'By the time I had finished the course I was really quite under-confident about my personal abilities ... It really does destroy your confidence because it makes you tear yourself apart and put yourself together again.... You have to do this when you are reflecting ... and then you have to repair yourself.'

Other nurses suggested that they had had problems coming to terms with the need to continually identify and analyse their feelings because this had a dominating effect on their lives.

> 'When you have got used to reflecting I don't think you can completely let go ... I don't think it is something you can switch off because it becomes a way of thinking, although it may not be to the same level as you did for your [course].

I don't think you ever lose the ability to learn from reflection and it becomes part of you and part of everyday life ... but I did remember a point of thinking "no, no get me away from all this reflection stuff, it's invading my life"...'

There was a range of personal interpretations and most of these could be traced back to the literature that had underpinned the course philosophy (George 1986). Throughout the year, all the nurses said they continued to be influenced by the reflective process that had been introduced to them during the course.

'I still reflect ... at the time you start during the course ... you think is this really necessary? But then you realise as you go on that it is a useful sort of thing.... [At first] you are doing it because it is part of your course ... and in doing it you think this is really worthwhile [and] you can see the purpose of it...'

Towards the end of the year all the nurses acknowledged some positive benefits of reflection and it was suggested that there had been a resurgence in this activity. From most of the accounts it appeared that nurses had begun to reflect 'on', if not 'in' action:

'I reflected about the whole situation a great deal. I [asked myself] if it ever happened again, would I do the same things? Would I say the same things? ... How would I approach that again? ... How would I improve it?'

'I reflect on how [the situation] went, whether it went well or not, how you would alter it subsequently, would you alter it, if so why?, if not why not? and how would you go about a similar situation again?'

Challenging the status quo: the influence of reflection

Nurses in the study suggested that a critical approach to their practice encouraged them to challenge the 'status quo' and that this distinguished them from nurses who had undertaken traditional training where reflection had not been a major component of the curriculum.

'Whenever a child goes home you think about how things have gone and if things have gone well and if things have gone ... badly ... you think about it and then try and change things ... [in the] old style of training people just accepted the status quo.'

It was also suggested that being in possession of a sound knowledge base and reflective skills gave them confidence to constructively challenge practice.

'If I am not happy about a certain way of doing something I'll go and read about it, get the research, talk to people and question things rather than just carry it out because I saw someone else doing it that way.' [Mary]

However, the nurses sometimes appeared to be reticent to do this and it was intimated that being taught to question or challenge was potentially uncomfortable because in the clinical area the staff nurse who challenges practice can be viewed as aggressive and radical.

'You have to learn ... that you can't question [everything] because it is not appropriate. You come up against a lot of barriers and if you start questioning things fences start to go up and you could be seen as someone who is aggressive and unhappy with things as they are ... It is harder questioning [practice] as a staff nurse because as a student people accept it but as a staff nurse [you are just seen as] radical...' [Nancy]

Reflection: a private contemplation

Several nurses described reflection as an informal, personal, solitary and subconscious process, suggesting that this way of thinking about practice had been internalised:

'[Reflection] is ... drummed into you for four years, it becomes ... a part of your thinking and rather than separate [ing] ... the reflective part of my brain [from] the rest of me. It sort of meshed together so I probably use it without realising it half the time.'

Often, they engaged in this activity on their own and offered examples of where they 'sat down at home' to reflect and work out the 'good and bad bits' of a situation. During this time they sometimes evaluated whether, in hindsight, their actions had been appropriate and they planned for the management of future similar situations.

'I actually sat down and worked out the good and bad bits of the day and the whole situation. It was helpful because it did prove to me that I did know what I was doing and I did have the skills and knowledge to handle the situation and I did do it correctly.'

'If I come home feeling I have had a stressful day or if l come home feeling very dissatisfied then I will use reflection as a way of coping with that ... and explore all the channels ... and try and get to the route of why I am feeling hacked off.'

Although initially reflection had been described as a solitary activity, as the year progressed the nurses began to reflect with other members of the team especially when debriefing after stressful situations and they appeared to derive support from this.

'At the time I was very angry and very upset and to use your word, "reflecting". Just thinking about it was the only way that I could come to terms with it. [I also] discussed it with other people and a lot of people felt upset about it so talking to each other and thrashing it out all helped.'

'The second time ... I knew the child better then and understood her needs. I tried to diffuse the whole situation and I tried to make it very fresh and new and to deal with it in a different way from the way we did before ... I tried to create a relaxed atmosphere ... and planned how the day went... That is reflection. It is self, looking at the way forward to actually make a situation different. It does work and having sat down to think about it I was more relaxed as well...'

Reflection as a means of integrating theory, research and practice

Most of the nurses acknowledged that, during the course, they had been taught to use the literature and research to provide a rationale for the care they were giving. They referred to the ways in which they had been taught to reflect on practice as instrumental in encouraging this integration. They contrasted themselves with colleagues who had undertaken the DipHE course and considered that they placed a greater value on research. There were many examples throughout the year of their attempts to use reflective practice to integrate research and theory within their practice.

'I quite often think of research based things whereas sometimes you work with people who just do things. [I feel I am] able to contribute ideas by talking to people about research.'

The role of reflection in encouraging self directed learning

Many of the nurses alluded to the fact that reflection had encouraged them to identify their learning needs, assess their own level of competence, examine their accountability and to articulate their concerns before taking on new responsibilities. They had a tendency to seek out the knowledge they needed before they embarked on new skills or confronted potentially difficult situations. This occurred despite their feeling that this sometimes created minor difficulties with their peers.

'The [other nurses] moan slightly at my accountability because I won't do anything unless I am one hundred percent sure . . . I think that is something the degree course has shown me is important.' [Barbara]

Their propensity towards being self directed increased towards the latter part of the year, especially when they considered expanding their roles in practice. They had an aptitude for learning new skills and a desire to continue their professional education.

'[Having done a degree course] you are quite quick to take new things on board . . . other . . . staff have commented on how quickly we seem to learn new skills. I think it is because we developed self-awareness and self-learning therefore we expect to say "right I want to give IVs" and then to go off and read about it. I make sure I get the support [I] need rather than waiting to be spoon-fed . . .'

Circumstances in which the nurses used reflection

Figure 8.1 shows the circumstances in which the nurses used reflection. During the year the nurses discussed specific events that they felt gave insight into the ways in which they engaged in elements of the reflective process.

'I think [reflection] has been instilled in you so much and . . . that is how I have improved over the time I have been qualified because I have continued to think through . . . critical incidents and all the things that have happened on the ward. . . . My assessment of the situation was that . . . perhaps this person felt a bit threatened by me. If they did, by me actually facing them and saying "What's your problem?" would only make matters worse. I decided to back off and allow them their space to set up their walls and their defences . . . I could have got really upset about it. I could have challenged her about it. I could have flown off the handle . . . but I was able to actually sit back and say "I feel this is going on, this is how I feel about it, this is how I am going to deal with it . . ." and . . . then to be able to say that worked well . . .' Also with patient care it's the same thing . . . it just happens. So I do think reflection has an influence.'

When 'reflecting' the nurses seemed to use a similar questioning approach and typical questions are identified in Figure 8.2. Figure 8.3 summarises the ways in which nurses described their use of reflection.

Discussion and conclusions

This chapter has presented some research findings in relation to the legacy of reflective practice. On the whole the nurses' descriptors of

Participant	Uses of reflection
Alison	To examine previous knowledge and experience to inform the introduction of proposed changes within the unit.
Barbara, Sandra	To improve organisation of the oncology admissions. To examine the experience of a child having an invasive procedure.
Alison, Barbara, Claire, James, Joanne	To assist in stress management or debriefing after a challenging shift, cardiac arrest.
Christine	To analyse the effectiveness of health education advice given to an adolescent following tonsillectomy.
Claire	To reconsider the management of a child who haemorrhaged. To explore the ethical and legal implications of discovering cocaine in a child's locker. To explore a solution to problems with communications between nurses and medical staff.
James	To manage a conflict with a colleague whilst co-ordinating the ward. Intervening in a challenging situation with a parent.
Joanne	To explore feelings when caring for a very sick child.
Mary	To explore the effectiveness of communication when caring for a child with a newly diagnosed cerebral tumour.

Fig. 8.1   Circumstances in which the nurses used reflection.

reflection mirrored those espoused in the literature (for example Schön 1987, Gibbs 1988). The lasting influence of reflection could be ascertained from the ways in which they discussed during the interviews the significant events arising from practice. There is evidence that when nurses are inaugurated into reflective practice during their educational programme it sometimes has a personal cost in terms of self-analysis and this supports the view of Burnard (1995). This may have accounted for the reluctance on the part of some of the nurses in this study to engage in the self analysis during the first few months following registration. In the longer term it could be argued that there is increasing evidence of the legacy of reflection, although they did not seem to examine their feelings to the same extent as they had on the course and there was a marked tendency to look back on past situations rather that to reflect in the middle of situations.

Alison	What did we do? What should we have done that we didn't do? How would we act differently, what could we do next time?
Barbara	What have I done? How could I do things better in the future? How can I change things?
Mary	Have I done the best that I could possibly do? Is there anything I could do differently next time?
Christine	What happened? Why did it happen? How can I change it? What was good, how can I do it again? What did I do before? How did I cope with this and if it worked before would I do it again?
Sandra	How does that make me feel? How does that make them feel? What went well? Did we work as a team? What were the good and bad aspects?

Fig. 8.2   Examples of questions the nurses typically asked during reflection.

All the nurses studied perceived that the course, and particularly reflection, continued to have an influence upon them throughout the year in several ways:

- in terms of the ways in which they thought about their practice and the extent to which they used research
- there was evidence that the reflective cycle (Gibbs 1988) was a useful tool to guide their systematic debriefing with their colleagues following stressful events
- there was an affiliation between reflection and the development of confidence and an acknowledgement of the synergy between competence, confidence, experience and reflection.

It has been demonstrated that there is a symbiotic relationship between competence and confidence and the first year of professional practice is characterised by a progression in both (Dearmun 1997b). An association between practice, reflection and the development of confidence has also been verified, supporting previous studies (Hallett 1997b; MacLeod 1996, Benner *et al.* 1996).

	Participants (initials only)									
	A	B	CH	CL	E	JA	JO	M	N	S
They thought about what they were about to do before they did it.						✓		✓	✓	✓
They thought about what they were doing while they were doing it.						✓		✓		✓
They looked back and thought about what they had done.			✓	✓	✓	✓		✓	✓	✓
They analysed situations in order to bring about changes or improvements in their future practice.		✓		✓	✓			✓	✓	✓
They balanced the positive and negative aspects of a situation.		✓		✓	✓			✓	✓	✓
They questioned and critically analysed situations, seeing them from different angles and perspectives in order to appreciate the whole.			✓	✓	✓	✓			✓	
They integrated their experience, theory or research into their practice.				✓	✓	✓			✓	✓
They examined their feelings.						✓				

Fig. 8.3 Ways nurses described their use of reflection.

Confidence comes with experience in the field, and this is contingent upon time to amass experience and reflect upon these experiences. It could be argued that, through reflection the nurses' knowledge and skills can be propagated and this heralds the increase in their confidence. Overall there is a suggestion that, rather than learning through formal contrived processes, experience seems to be gained from 'taking the plunge', or 'being thrown in at the deep end' and using reflection to handle traumatic or demanding situations successfully (Dearmun 1997b). An acknowledgement of this has implications for the pacing of experience for new practitioners but it appears that reflective skills are tools with which they can judge their own capabilities accurately and enlist the support they need.

In terms of the development of confidence, each of the nurses had a unique experience but their progress followed an analogous sequence that was affected by similar contextual influences. The rate at which they reached particular milestones was dictated by the responsibilities that they had been allowed to assume, or had been given, and the ways in which they coped with these. Acceding that confidence was born of experience and was accelerated following the successful handling of demanding experiences, the submission is made that neophyte nurses who are given responsibility progress more quickly than those nurses who are over protected. Rather than contributing to reality shock, being given the authority to work independently, making decisions, or being left in demanding situations was instrumental in creating a surge in confidence. It is also suggested that the increase in the nurses' confidence altered their perceptions of stressful and challenging events. Perhaps, given this, the inclusion of reflection in the nurses' repertoire of coping strategies, (Schön 1991) for these events is even more pertinent.

Perhaps, as a result of being in situations where they had had to implement care for children with a range of acuity and dependency, by the end of their first year most nurses had developed a secure belief in their own abilities, and as such, were able to give support to the parents, supervise less experienced colleagues and mentor student nurses. The fact that a year after graduation nurses felt sufficiently competent and confident to pass on their knowledge and skills to others may be testament to their progress and development and possibly their reflective skills.

Limitations of the study

The characteristics identified in this study may be entirely a feature of this particular cohort of graduate nurses and further research is required in order to substantiate the claim made. Although the evidence is not generalisable, there are indications that besides experience and being given responsibilities, having the skills to reflect upon these experiences and receiving positive and constructive comments on work performance are also pivotal to the development of confidence.

The research process used to elicit the nurses' views demanded retrospective accounts and this may have accentuated the proclivity to look back and report on situations that had occurred and embellish them (Reece Jones 1995), thus, making it impossible to capture the extent to which the nurses engaged in reflection in the midst of situations (Newell 1992, Greenwood 1993).

It may be concluded that, although the value of reflection was acknowledged by the nurses, they commonly referred to it as a subconscious activity. This may indicate one of two positions: either it had become an integral part of their thought processes and thus, it was tacit in their practice. Or that they could not extrapolate examples of reflection because they did not really engage in this activity, and their disposition to reflect upon their practice may have remained dormant but for prompting by the interviews. The problems of social desirability have been well recognised (Patton 1990) and despite attempts to build up trust with the participants and emphasise the confidential and non-judgemental nature of the enquiry, it is possible that the nurses accentuated practices, traits and made comments that they believed would be valued and acceptable (Patton 1990, Brink 1991).

It appears that assessing a practitioner's spontaneous use of reflection is fraught with difficulty and caution should be exercised before drawing unequivocal conclusions that the process of reflection influences a nurse's practice after qualifying. Further still that it has a direct effect upon patient care; an aspect of reflection that has yet to receive research attention. Nevertheless these practitioners continued to recognise the structured analytical approach referred to as reflection and so to an extent the optimism among the educators that nurses from the BA (Hons) course would continue to analyse incidents arising from practice was founded. In this way a tendency to learn from experience was enduring and it could be argued that, by continuing to evaluate their emerging knowledge and skills and analysing their performance, nurses improve the quality of their practice.

References

Argyris, C. & Schön, D. (1974) *Theory in Practice: Increasing Professional Effectiveness*, Addison Wesley, Reading.

Atkins, S. & Murphy, K. (1993) Reflection: a review of the literature. *Journal of Advanced Nursing*, **18**, 1188–92.

Bassett, C. (1993) Socialisation of student nurses into the qualified nurse role. *British Journal of Nursing*, **2** (3), 179–82.

Benner, P. (1984) *From Novice to Expert: Excellence and Power in Clinical Nursing*, Addison Wesley, Menlo Park, California.

Benner, P. & Tanner, C.A. (1987) Clinical judgement: how nurses use intuition. *American Journal of Nursing*, **1**, 23–31.

Benner, P., Tanner, C.A. & Chesla, C.A. (1996). *Expertise in Nursing Practice: Caring, Clinical Judgement and Ethics*, Springer Publishing.

Boud, D., Keogh, R. & Walker, D. (1985) *Reflection: Turning Experience into Learning*, Kogan Page, London; Nichols Pub Co., New York.

Brink, P.J. (1991) Issues of reliability and validity. In Morse, J.M. (ed.) *Qualitative Nursing Research: A Contemporary Dialogue*, Sage Publications Ltd, London.

Burnard, P. (1995) Nurse educators' perceptions of reflection and reflective practice: a report of a descriptive study. *Journal of Advanced Nursing*, **21**, 1167–74.

Burns, S. (1992) Grading practice. *Nursing Times* **88** (1), 40–42.

Dearmun, A.K. (1996) Reflection: continuing education series. *Paediatric Nursing*, **8** (3), 30–33.

Dearmun, A.K. (1997a) *The Perceptions of Newly Qualified Children's Nurses about their First Year of Professional Practice*, Reading University, Unpublished PhD Thesis.

Dearmun, A.K. (1997b) Assessing practice at degree level. *Paediatric Nursing*, **9** (1), 25–9.

Dearmun, A.K. (1998) Perceptions of job stress. *Journal of Child Health Nursing*, **2** (3), 132–7.

Dewey, J. (1933) *How We Think*, D.C. Heath, Boston.

Dewey, J. (1938) *Experience and Education*, Macmillan, London.

Entwhistle, N. & Ramsden, P. (1983) *Understanding Student Learning*, Croom, London.

George, P. (1986) *The Nurse as a Reflective Practitioner*, Unpublished paper, Department of Social Studies Oxford Polytechnic, Oxford.

Glaser, B.G. & Strauss, A.L. (1966) The purpose and credibility of qualitative research. *Nursing Research*, **15** (1), 56–61.

Morse, J. (1991) (ed.) *Qualitative Nursing Research: A Contemporary Dialogue*, Sage Publications (revised edn), London.

Gibbs, G. (1988) *Learning by Doing: A Guide to Teaching and Learning Methods*, Further Education Unit, Oxford Polytechnic, Oxford.

Greenwood, J. (1993) Reflective practice: a critique of the work of Argyris and Schön. *Journal of Advanced Nursing*, **19**, 1183–87.

Haddock, J. & Bassett, C. (1997) Nurses' perceptions of reflective practice. *Nursing Standard*, **11** (32), 39–41.

Hallett, C. (1997a) Pragmatism and Project 2000: the relevance of Dewey's theory of experimentalism to nursing education. *Journal of Advanced Nursing*, **26**, 1229–234.

Hallett, C. (1997b) Learning through reflection in the community: the relevance of Schön's theories of coaching to nursing education. *International Journal of Nursing Studies*, **34** (2), 103–110.

Hallett, C.E., Williams, A. & Butterworth, T. (1996) The learning career in the community setting: a phenomenological study of a Project 2000 placement. *Journal of Advanced Nursing*, **23** (3), 578–86.

Harding, R. (1997) Reflections on family centred care. *Paediatric Nursing*, **9** (9), 19–21.

Holloway, I.M. & Penson, J. (1987) Nurse education as social control. *Nurse Education Today* **7**, 235–41.

Jarvis, P. (1992) Reflective practice and nursing. *Nurse Education Today*, **12** (2), 174–81.

James, C.R. & Clarke, B.A. (1994) Reflective practice in nursing: issues and implications for nurse education. *Nurse Education Today*, **14**, 82–90.

Johns, C. (1994) Guided reflection. In Palmer, A., Burns, S. & Bulman, C. (eds) *Reflective Practice in Nursing*, Blackwell Scientific Publications, Oxford.

Kohner, N. (1994) *Clinical Supervision: An Executive Summary*, Kings Fund Centre, London.

Kolb, D.A. (1984) *Experimental Learning*, Prentice Hall, New Jersey.

Kramer, M. (1968) Role models, role conceptions and role deprivation. *Nursing Research*, **17** (2), 115–20.

Kramer, M. (1974) *Reality Shock: Why Nurses Leave the Profession*, Mosby Co., St Louis.

Kramer, M. (1985) Why does reality shock continue? In McCloskey, J. & Grace, J. (eds) *Current Issues in Nursing*,Blackwell Scientific Publications, Boston.

Lamond, N. (1974) *Becoming a Nurse: The Registered Nurse's View of General Student Nurse Education*, RCN, London.

Lowe, P.B. & Kerr, C.M. (1998) Learning by reflection: the effect on educational outcomes. *Journal of Advanced Nursing*, **27**, 1030–33.

MacLeod, M.L.P. (1996) *Practising Nursing – Becoming Experienced*, Churchill Livingstone, London.

McCaugherty, D. (1991) The use of a teaching model to promote reflection and the experiential integration of yheory and practice in first year student nurses: an action research study. *Journal of Advanced Nursing*, **16** (3), 534–543.

Mezirow, J. (1981) A critical theory of adult learning and education. *Adult Education*, **32** (1), 3–24.

Newell, R. (1992) Anxiety, accuracy and reflection: the limits of professional development. *Journal of Advanced Nursing*, **17**, 1326–33.

NHSME (1997) *The New NHS – Modern and Dependable.*

NHSME (1998) *A First Class Service: Quality in the NHS.*

Palmer, A., Burns, S. & Bulman, C. (1994) *Reflective Practice in Nursing: The Growth of the Professional Practitioner*, Blackwell Scientific Publications, London.

Patton, M.Q. (1990) *Qualitative Evaluation and Research Methods*, Sage (second edn), London.

Pierson, W. (1998) Reflection and nursing education. *Journal of Advanced Nursing*, **27**, 165–70.

Powell, J. (1989) The reflective practitioner in nursing. *Journal of Advanced Nursing*, **14**, 824–32.

Reece Jones, P. (1995) Hindsight bias in reflective practice: an empirical investigation. *Journal of Advanced Nursing*, **21**, 783–8.

Richardson, G. Maltby, H. (1995) Reflection-on-practice: enhancing student learning. *Journal of Advanced Nursing*, **22**, 235-42.

Rolfe, G. (1997) Beyond expertise: theory, practice and the reflective practitioner. *Journal of Clinical Nursing*, **6**, 93–97.

Schön, D. (1983) *The Reflective Practitioner: How Professionals Think in Action*, Temple Smith, London.

Schön, D. (1987) *Educating the Reflective Practitioner*, Jossey Bass, San Francisco.

Schön, D (1991) *The Reflective Practitioner*, second edn, Jossey Bass, San Francisco.

Simpson, I.H. (1979) *From Student to Nurse: A Longitudinal Study of Socialisation*, Cambridge University Press, London.

Van Manen, M. (1991) Reflectivity and the pedagogical moment: the normativity of pedagogical thinking and acting. *Journal of Curriculum Studies*, **23** (6), 507–536.

Wooton, S.J. (1997) The reflective process as a tool for learning: a personal account. *Paediatric Nursing*, **9** (2), 6–8.

Chapter 9
Exemplars of Reflection: A chance to Learn through the Inspiration of Others

Introduction

It has become evident through my own thinking and learning about reflection that the experience of others using the reflective process can be an inspiration to those that are just starting out on their reflective journey. I hope that this chapter will enable you to consider the work of others in a way that may inspire you to try out reflection for yourself. As you no doubt will have discovered from previous chapters, reflection is not always an easy journey and there is a possibility that you may feel disheartened by some of the more articulate exemplars illustrated in this chapter. Rest assured however that every contributor has had to begin their own journey somewhere. Each has survived the experience, with the appreciation that the ability to learn from experience has strengthened them as practitioners. You have the benefit of sharing in their efforts. A little bit of inspiration here may be enough to get you started on your own reflective journey, and using some of the frameworks and practical tips for reflection.

Why bother to reflect at all?

If human beings did not possess the ability to be thoughtful about the problems of life, one could question whether we, for instance, would ever have harnessed the benefits of fire or invented the wheel. Those cynics among you will no doubt declare at this point that the trouble with human beings is that sometimes they think too much and do not develop and learn from this great capacity.

It is at this stage that the ability to reflect rather than simply be thoughtful is worth dwelling on. Jarvis (1992) suggests that reflection is not just thoughtful practice but a learning experience. Just as in life, nursing involves situations that are complex and if we are to understand nursing and ourselves as nurses, we need to try and make sense of the complexity. The trouble with nursing as with life in general is that it is dynamic, constantly changing, challenging, frustrating and exciting often all at the same time. Therefore, as practitioners of nursing it is impossible to declare that we have nursing 'in the bag'; that we know all there is to know or that we have reached a final understanding of practice.

However, it is possible to explore ourselves as professionals, by reflecting on our experiences, in order to develop our self awareness and ability to self evaluate. This reflective approach is typified by growth and learning rather than the reliance on ritual and automatic pilot to get us through the day (Street 1991, Saylor 1990, Schon 1983). Indeed Jarvis (1992) advocates the need for reflective practice since nurses are dealing with people, who because of their individual nature require us to be responsive and reflective, instead of simply carrying out routine, ritual and presumption. In order to be effective in practice there is a requirement to be purposeful and goal directed (Street 1991), thus reflection cannot just be concerned with understanding but must also include changing practice (Driscoll 1994). You will certainly be able to detect personal considerations of change and development in the exemplars that follow. It is also possible that theory development arising from practice could emerge as nurses acquire a more reflective way of practising nursing, giving them the insight to 'grow' nursing theory from practice itself.

A word of caution is justified at this point. I believe that reflection could offer most of us a route toward exploring our ability to be therapeutic in our practice. This can only be achieved by the fostering of self awareness and an ability to be constructively critical in order to facilitate positive change. We may pay a price for this however, even though it could be one that is worthwhile in the long run, since reflection is not always comfortable (Saylor 1990, Carr 1996). This is a point amply illustrated in the exemplars that follow. Reflection will force us to face incongruity and uncomfortable facts about nursing, the organisations we work in and ourselves. One must consider both the positive and negative aspects before embarking on a reflective pathway, and educationalists introducing reflection as part of a curriculum must be aware of this and need carefully to consider the support required for such an approach (James & Clarke 1994).

You will be able to identify the concepts outlined above throughout the exemplars in the rest of the chapter:

- to appreciate that situations in nursing can be complex
- to resolve to try and understand what nursing is about
- to strive to be self aware and to self evaluate
- to question routine and ritualisation
- to develop and challenge current practice.

Helping you to start

Many of the tips mentioned below will seem familiar, as they will have been covered in different contexts throughout the book. They are represented here in a summarised form as they give you the chance to consider what you need to work on at a glance, rather than necessarily needing to plough through the book, except where you may require further detail. Consequently the following may be worth considering.

Use a framework to help you to reflect

Four references to frameworks are given starting on page 178. They are illustrative of the type of tools that qualified and unqualified nurses have used in order to help them with their reflection.

Find someone with whom to reflect

A colleague, mentor or supervisor can provide a sounding board, open up different perspectives and provide support and guidance. It is helpful to find someone who already has experience of using reflection and who is someone that you trust, if you are to share and explore your experiences and feelings. The role of mentor is explored further in Chapter 4; similarly the role of the clinical supervisor is explored in Chapter 5. You may find it useful to revisit these chapters when you are considering setting up a relationship with a mentor or supervisor. Managers and educationalists would also benefit from these chapters when considering reflection as a strategy for learning about practice.

Keeping a reflective journal or diary

Keeping a regular diary is an extremely useful tip, since the memory of events can fade quickly even for those with the most photographic of memories (Newell 1992). You may find it helpful to build up a personal repertoire of experience in your diary which you will be able to use to reflect back on and draw from, as you gain in experience. It is worth setting aside time to write in your diary in a form that feels comfortable for you. Using an attractively bound file or book in which to record your reflections may promote your motivation to write. Johns (1994) suggests splitting each page; using the left hand side to write up your diary and the right hand side for further reflections, analysis and notes. He suggests writing down exactly what is said: sentences and key phrases, in order to capture the situation. He also recommends aiming to reflect on both problematic and satisfying experiences. You may wish to record experiences concerning your own patients or situations that seemed dramatic or special in practice. However, it is possible to miss out on seemingly routine or mediocre events which on reflection could prove to be useful learning experiences.

Johns also suggests that openness and honesty is an integral part of good diary keeping; however, it is essential to preserve the anonymity and confidentiality of clients even if your diary is private (Hargreaves 1997). There is no doubt from my own experience that diary keeping requires motivation and commitment; some people find it easier to do than others. The most important thing is to find a method of recording your experiences that works for you.

Educationalists should be aware of the support and guidance needed if diary keeping or journal writing is to be advocated as part of learning about practice. I believe they also need to consider carefully the issue of privacy and students' diaries and how writing about experience is shared and supported if students are asked to keep journals as part of their academic assessment. The work of Burnard (1991), Hargreaves (1997), Heinrich (1992), Newell (1992), Paterson (1995), Richardson & Maltby (1995), Shields (1995), and Wellard & Bethune (1996) among others are worthy of analysis before students are exposed to the rigours of diary or journal keeping. Chapter 3 in this book by Pam Sharp and Cath Davies also considers the issues of diary keeping within the context of the assessment and evaluation of reflection.

Reading the literature

We hope that this book will provide you with some useful background on reflection. It is important that you understand the concepts involved and have a clear idea of what you personally might find helpful in starting to reflect. Sue Atkins' chapter, Chapter 2, provides some useful tips and theoretical background to the attributes necessary for true reflection and Mary FitzGerald and Ysanne Chapman's chapter, Chapter 1, explores the literature on reflection. Additionally, Chapter 6, which looks at the student's perspectives, provides some useful insights from students on using literature to build on your analysis of practice.

Having the courage to change and/or challenge

As mentioned previously, reflection can be painful as well as enlightening, often bringing things to conscious thought that need to be dealt with. This is not easy to deal with and requires the support of a good mentor/supervisor. Importantly Hargreaves (1997) warns of the potential vulnerability of students exposed to reflection and advocates the need for support and ethical direction from educationalists. Of course it is helpful if you work in an environment where positive change and constructive challenge are welcomed in the workplace, it is easier then to be brave and voice your reflections on practice (Cullingford 1991). If you are not in such a position you need to seek out supportive and facilitative networks, before you set off on a reflective pathway.

A framework for reflection

For someone filled with enthusiasm to begin to reflect, the dilemma of where to start can rapidly spring to mind. Consequently, I have included suggestions below for use as frameworks, for going about the business of reflection. It may be that you feel comfortable with one particular framework and opt to use it every time you reflect. It is not essential to use a framework, some practitioners choose not to. The suggestions here are not exhaustive and there are many more ideas available in the literature, for example the work of Mezirow (1981), Burnard (1991), Boud, Keogh & Walker (1985), and Driscoll (1994) all provide help for the reflective practitioner.

Since reflection is not a static process but a dynamic one it is appropriate to include a framework with an overt cyclical approach. The reflective framework illustrated in Figure 4.2 (page 83) is adapted from a framework for experiential learning and guides you through a series of questions, in order to provide structure when reflecting on an experience. You can begin at the top of the cycle asking the question, 'What happened?' and then progress around the cycle in order to explore an experience in practice and to guide the reflective process.

Johns' (1995b) model of structured learning is composed of a series of questions helping the reflective practitioner to tune into an experience and provide structure and meaning to the process of reflection. It has emerged through Chris Johns' extensive work through which practitioners explored their experiences in supervision (Johns 1993, 1994, 1995a, 1995b).

Goodman (1984) distinguishes three levels of reflection that the reflective practitioner may achieve. These levels could serve as a broad guide for you and for teachers in assessing the quality and depth of reflective work. In fact, Goodman's work amongst others informs the assessment of reflective work at Oxford Brookes University.

Write a description of the experience.

Cue questions

Aesthetics:	What was I trying to achieve?
	Why did I respond as I did?
	What were the consequences of that for the patient, others, myself?
	How was this person feeling? (or these persons?)
	How did I know this?
Personal:	How did I feel in this situation?
	What internal factors were influencing me?
Ethics:	How did my actions match my beliefs?
	What factors made me act in incongruent ways?
Empirics:	What knowledge did or should have informed me?
Reflexivity:	How does this connect with previous experiences?
	Could I handle this better in similar situations?
	What would be the consequences of alternative actions for:
	the patient?
	others?
	myself?
	How do I *now* feel about this experience?
	Can I support myself and others better as a consequence?
	Has this changed my ways of knowing?

Fig. 9.1   A model of structured reflection (10th version) (Johns 1995b, p.227)

1st Level
Reflection to reach given objectives: Criteria for reflection are limited to technocratic issues of efficiency, effectiveness and accountability.

2nd Level
Reflection on the relationship between principles and practice: There is an assessment of the implications and consequences of actions and beliefs as well as the underlying rationale for practice.

3rd level
Reflection which besides the above incorporates ethical and political concerns: Issues of justice and emancipation enter deliberations over the value of professional goals and practice and the practitioner makes links between the setting of everyday practice and broader social structure and forces.

Fig. 9.2   Goodman's levels of reflection (Goodman 1984).

A final framework has been chosen which poses a series of questions for you to work through. It emerged from the experiences of Sarah Stephenson, who wrote in the first edition of this book. She was immersed in reflection throughout her pre-registration, undergraduate studies, and her framework is worth sharing with others (Figure 9.3).

> **Choose a situation from your placement; ask yourself...**
> - What was my role in this situation?
> - Did I feel comfortable or uncomfortable? Why?
> - What actions did I take?
> - How did I and others act?
> - Was it appropriate?
> - How could I have improved the situation for myself, the patient, my mentor?
> - What can I change in future?
> - Do I feel as if I have learnt anything new about myself?
> - Did I expect anything different to happen? What and why?
> - Has it changed my way of thinking in any way?
> - What knowledge from theory and research can I apply to this situation?
> - What broader issues, for example ethical, political or social, arise from this situation?
> - What do I think about these broader issues?

Fig. 9.3 A student's own framework for reflection (Taken from Stephenson 1994, pp. 56–7).

Exemplars from practice

The following exemplars of reflection are contributions from a wide range of nurses and a midwifery student. They include the work of both qualified nurses and students and span through undergraduate to postgraduate work. These examples are presented as written by the contributors, each contributor has used pseudonyms for people and places as appropriate. The content of the exemplars has not been altered, except where the need for brevity has prevailed. They simply serve to illustrate practitioners reflecting on their practice. Questions are included among the exemplars to challenge the reader and highlight points for you to consider in developing your reflective skills.

Exemplar 1

This exemplar is taken from the learning contract of an undergraduate pre-registration student in the paediatric field of nursing.

'I am still aware that I do assume parents will do all the care for their child in hospital, I particularly became aware of this when admitting children with special needs. Amy was a three year old child with a large haemangioma which spread over one side of her face and neck. She had a permanent tracheostomy tube in situ and was therefore unable to communicate in words. Her parents were experts in her care that consisted of communicating with a simplified version of the Makaton vocabulary, operating the portable suction equipment and administering drugs through a gastrostomy tube. When admitting Amy I was anxious to be aware of all her needs and went through her assessment slowly with her parents.

'When I arrived at the section about parental participation I heard myself say, "I assume you want to carry out all of Amy's care while she is here...?" I used that dreaded word!! Her mother said that she would, although looked more resigned to it than willing, I tried immediately to correct myself by saying that we were there to help and relieve her if she was in need of a rest, but I realised the damage had already been done. I reflected on my reasons for asking this question, I wondered if perhaps subconsciously I was too nervous about carrying out the care myself, because I was unfamiliar with it. If so my approach of shying away from the challenge was wrong. I know that with support and guidance from the parents and my mentor, I am capable of caring for a child with complex needs like Amy's and it would only have served to reassure me of my competence. I also considered the possibility that I asked this question because I felt that Amy's parents would only feel reassured about her care if they continued to do it themselves. Coyne (1995) [student did not include reference] found that reasons for parents participating in care were concern about relinquishing care to strangers and a sense of parental duty, which seems to suggest being pressured into care. I felt that I had perhaps pressured Amy's parents into agreeing to this participation when in fact they may have been glad of a well deserved rest by handing the care to professionals.'

Questions

- How well do you think the student has managed to describe the situation?
- Can you decide where her description ends and where her process of reflection begins?
- Are you able to pick out her feelings about this particular incident?
- Work your way through the questions posed in Stephenson's framework. Can you see how the student may have addressed some of these? What else could the student have included in her reflection?

Exemplar 2

This exemplar is the work of an undergraduate pre-registration, North American exchange student (adult field). She reflects on the intricacies of caring for an unconscious patient and his family.

'On several occasions I provided care for HY, a 45-year old man who was admitted to the ward after hitting his head. On the same day a craniotomy was performed to evacuate a subdural haematoma. HY had been non-responsive since that time except for the slight twitching of his mouth and flexion of his left leg. I assessed him according to the Glasgow scale that indicates level of consciousness and confirmed a score of three, the same score that a dead person would receive (no response to questions of orientation, no response to commands, no opening of the eyes in response to communication or pain). The Glasgow coma scale tests the patient's ability in each of the following areas: eye opening, motor response and verbal response (Powell 1994, p. 23, Lindsay *et al.* 1991). HY received the minimum possible score of three, which suggests "a very serious injury and little likelihood of total recovery" (Powell 1994, p. 23). His state was described as "flat" suggesting no spontaneous movement or interaction. HY breathes on his own and that combined with the movement of his mouth gives the impression that he is merely sleeping.'

- Is the above description or reflection?

'As K and I suctioned his tracheostomy, performed a range of motion exercises and repositioned him to prevent bed sores, I was curious to know what exactly had brought him to this state and was there any chance of recovery? After all he was breathing on his own (which was virtually the only response distinguishing him from a deceased person) and appeared to be merely sleeping. While I cared for HY I kept feeling he might open his eyes every time he twitched his mouth. I felt a mixture of sadness at his present condition and hope that he might recover.'

- What stage in the reflective cycle (Gibbs 1988) is the student in now?

'HY's family continues to have faith that he will recover from his present state. He recovered from a year-long coma before this episode and they believed he might recover again. The power of their conviction is based on strong evidence and in my opinion cannot be argued with. Yet this belief may have affected my care in that I kept looking for signs of recovery instead of remaining objective. I have learned from my co-mentor that HY lost his family, his job and essentially his life during that year. He drank excessively and spoke harshly with his mother each night, to the point that his 95-year old mother took a blanket and sat on the porch each time he entered the back door to avoid the confrontations. She turns out to be the strongest advocator in doing the most for HY's condition, and the rest of his family also rallies behind him. In hearing a little about HY's history, I thought about the assumptions I had made about him and other patients. As a nursing student who very rarely cares for the same patient twice, I know very little about each patient as an individual. When I heard of HY's recovery from the first coma I felt sympathy for him and his family. It appeared that they supported him a great deal from the pictures and cards in his room, yet I was informed that they hadn't spoken to him much since the last time. I had already envisioned this warm family (and I am not saying that they aren't or couldn't be warm) who had suffered a great deal, celebrated, and now were suffering again. I also envisioned a kind-hearted father, husband and son who (unfairly?) has this condition. I can remember myself thinking that he doesn't deserve it. Yet with this new piece of news, my picture of him is more realistic. Do I think he deserves his present state? No! But I am now questioning my attitude towards patients and their illnesses.'

- How has the student's analysis of the situation developed?

'It is important to acknowledge the existence of the comatose patient by talking to them; withholding verbal conversation only emphasises the perception of them being dead (La Puma *et al.* 1988, p. 21). This was exemplified by K who talks to HY, telling him what she is doing and generally making small talk as she did with other patients. Her professional yet compassionate manner reinforces the fact that regardless of injury, illness or deficit, HY remains someone who deserves respect and effective care. This attitude is also emphasised by the fact that the door is closed during any procedure performed, even changing his feed. I can now appreciate the fact that biases, that declare some groups to be more worthy or deserving of services than others lead to gross inequities and must be avoided. (Wright 1982, p. 34).'

- How do you think the student uses the literature to inform reflection about her practice?

Exemplar 3

This exemplar is the work of an undergraduate, pre-registration, adult field student working in a medical unit; reflecting on her first experiences of admitting and assessing a patient.

'Patients are unlikely to want to be cared for by nurses who appear to lack competence or confidence; this may even enhance their fears and anxieties (French 1979). I have sat in a relaxed open posture and viewed patient's assessments on admission as "chats" where I get to know the patient a bit more and by conversing casually the patients get to know me and get the feel of the hospital.

On one incident when I was having such a chat with a patient he was at first very reserved as though he was sussing me out and I could see he was anxious about being in hospital. I recognised this and so decided to chat freely for a while, revealing parts of my own personality before asking the questions related to the assessment. I was striving to get over the uniform barrier. After a short while of chatting I feel he began to warm to me as his posture relaxed, his previously folded arms were gently placed in his lap and he extended his closed short answers to more detailed answers and even started asking me questions, such as about my training. This encouraged me as inside I was feeling a little nervous – that being my first admission.'

- What are your thoughts on the levels of reflection as described by Goodman (1984) that may be seen here?
- Taking into account your level of experience, what else may you have reflected on in a similar situation?

Exemplar 4

An undergraduate, pre-registration, adult field student reflecting on the issues to do with dependency and the promotion of self care.

'Another effect on hospitalisation is the dependency on care. It is important for nurses to be careful not to do everything for the patient and that they must promote self care. It can be easy when watching a patient, for example slowly reach for their slippers, for the nurse to say "oh, I'll get those for you", to stop the patient struggling and to save time. This can be seen as the nurse being nice and kind but the nurse would not be thinking of the patient's real needs.'

- What are your thoughts on the level of reflection here? (see Goodman)

'I have been in such a situation where I saw a patient struggle to reach her slippers, ready to walk to the bathroom and I felt very tempted to reach for them myself, so I had to stop myself. The patient needed to be able to care for herself in this way. She was perfectly able to carry out this task – just a little slower than perhaps I would. If I had done it for her then the patient may feel that I was taking away her independence or she may have started to become dependent on the nursing staff. One way of describing this may be pyjama-induced paralysis – when a patient comes into hospital they expect to put on their pyjamas get into bed and adopt a certain patient role. Parsons (1951) cited in Jones and Jones (1975) identifies that when someone feels unwell to the extent of seeking professional attention they require sick status and consequently adopt the sick role. There are four aspects to the sick role: the patient is exempted from normal responsibilities, the patient is not responsible for his illness and can make claims on others for assistance, the patient must want to get well, the patient must seek professional advice and co-operate with the treatment (Taylor & Field 1993).'

- How well does the student use the literature to develop her reflection?
- Can you relate extracts from this exemplar to the reflective cycle? (Gibbs)

Exemplar 5

Written by a final year direct entry, undergraduate midwifery student. The student reflects on the cultural and communication issues that surround her post-natal care for an Asian woman and her family.

'Breastfeeding seems to be a confusing issue for midwives caring for Muslim women. One of the cultural "barriers" is that many Muslim women view colostrum as unclean or like pus. I am told that some women coming from such a belief system do find out about the benefits of colostrum and go on to feed their babies from birth.

Yasmin is originally from Bangladesh, she married and came to England a short time ago and does not speak any English. When I came to her house for her post-natal check, I mistook her sister-in-law for the new mother, because she answered all my questions and was holding the baby. She even went to get the notes for me and showed me how much bottle milk the baby had taken that day. Yasmin eventually came down the stairs and we all laughed at my mistake, but the situation was tinted with the realisation that there was a cultural gap between us which meant that we could not understand each other, and this is why this had happened.

Yasmin said that she was fine, her husband said she was fine and so did her sister-in-law. They smiled and wondered why I had come there at all. Yasmin kept rubbing her breasts and when I asked if they were sore, she said no. When I asked if she had pain, she said, "yes very painful" I found out that she had become very engorged. Again the language barrier was glaringly apparent. We went upstairs, I looked at her breasts and I asked her repeatedly about the baby's feeding: how much breast, how much bottle? Did she want to breast feed or bottle feed? I was confused because I was not sure if she was bottle feeding as well as breast feeding until the true milk had come in, in which case I needed to make sure that she knew how to breastfeed well (to prevent mastitis and further engorgement). If she really wanted to bottle feed I needed to tell her how to reduce engorgement by not stimulating her breasts. It was very difficult to try and explain supply and demand to her. I was very confused and so was she. She told me through her sister-in-law translating that she wanted to breastfeed. So we set to work helping her to express some milk so that she could feed the baby and I could watch (she had already tried it once but was too engorged). After we had expressed for some time, I asked the same question again. This time the reply was that she was going to bottle feed. It was a struggle in this situation to try and provide optimum care. I realised just how vital the information from the woman is – how much women teach me about what they need from me.'

- What practice issues have highlighted this realisation for the student? How do you think her reflection has helped her to reach this conclusion?

'In this situation quality care was difficult to achieve, though I felt I made the best of a perplexing situation by persevering with questions where I was not sure of Yasmin's needs or decisions. I was sensitive towards Yasmin's feelings, trying to pick up cues from her that might guide me to a better understanding of her situation. I sensed that she needed support and guidance, that she had received no acknowledgment of her situation because of the language and culture barriers, which meant that we (midwives) could not understand her predicament.

'I made sure I documented my confusion in the careplan, and communicated with the group midwives about it, because I knew that it was beyond my limitations to really help Yasmin. This was partly due to communication difficulties and partly due to my inexperience. I wanted to make sure that Yasmin had good continuity of care with feeding her baby because I felt that it was creating emotional as well as psychological problems for her. She looked pale and did not smile or respond readily to questions. I wondered if I should send her to the breastfeeding counsellor, who I have used for a number of women this term, I feel that they need more support and continuity and someone with more experience than myself. I felt so powerless to help Yasmin in this situation. The communication barrier isolated us from one another and made discussing seemingly simple issues – such as the presence of breast pain, difficult and clouded by doubt. I wasn't even sure whether her replies were really the answers to my questions. However it was good in that I felt that I had supported her as well as I could, and I think she knew this. I drew pictures for her about positioning for breastfeeding and I made sure I repeated this to her husband and sister-in-law. Despite the difficulty with the feeding, the actual feeling – the atmosphere between us was positive and warm. I found being with them interesting and enjoyable and they seemed to trust me.'

- What positive and negative factors has the student been able to identify in this situation?
- Can you identify how the student has moved around the reflective cycle? (Gibbs)

'Midwifery practice is never going to be perfect, and we cannot hope to meet all women's needs all the time. Yasmin's needs were beyond my control, and to solve the problems would need a commitment of resources from local councils and hospital trusts to supply translators and written material for women with poor English skills. There are some things that I personally can do however. I have contacted an Urdu teacher so that she can translate a list of some basic midwifery words in Urdu for our use. This can be given to various units and other students for use on occasions when they might be looking after a woman who only speaks Urdu. This is just a token, but it could make a difference to some women's care. The same could be done in Chinese, Hindi, Bengali and other languages.'

- Look at Johns' model of structured reflection and try to work out how the student has progressed through this.

Exemplar 6

Written by a post-registration diploma student working in a critical care setting. Here she reflects on the issues connected with body image while caring for a women recovering from multiple injuries.

'I get up in the morning and look in the mirror and I have to say, am not usually happy with what I see. Too fat, too spotty, grey hair, the list could be endless. This shows that I on occasion have a problem with my body image. Schilder (1935) cited in Price (1990) defines body image as the picture of our body that we form in our mind; the way our body appears to ourselves. Simply put then, body image is the way we see ourselves. Perhaps I am unhappy with my body image, because obviously it evolves throughout life? Cronan (1993) suggests that body image problems arise naturally within the aging process because of conflicts between feelings and looks. I still feel inside a lot of the time as I did at 22, 23 – same moral values, beliefs, sense of fun – so I feel young but I look everyday at my 29 years - what a conflict. Society also puts pressure on your body image for example you only have to look at the media to see that good looking equals thin. Where is the room for the world's fat, birth-marked and teeth-braced people? Salter (1988) agrees suggesting that society exerts great pressure on us to comply with a certain image. While Cronan specifies fashion, mass media, socialisation and peer pressure as factors affecting body image formation, I have problems accepting my body image which is "normal", but will this knowledge help me address the problems of people with altered body image?'

- What feel do you get for this practitioner's sense of self awareness?

'What is altered body image? Wright (1986) suggests that any change in appearance or function of any part of our body threatens our body image. This change does not have to be obvious scarring or disfigurement. This is why I have chosen this objective. Every patient on the unit will have experienced some change in function that will affect how they feel about themselves. I want to develop an insight into what I can do to help and assist them come to terms with this change.

'K was a 40-year old lady who had been admitted to the ward with multiple injuries from ITU. All her injuries were fixed but she required split skin grafts to her left leg ...

'As K's condition improved she became aware of the physical aspect of altered body image. Dewing (1989) suggests that body image is composed of two components – the physical and the psychological. As will be revealed K had many psychological barriers to acceptance of her physical disabilities. Awareness of the skin grafts came only the first time they were dressed. When I began to take the dressings down, I explained that the grafts would look very red and raw, and that if she didn't want to look at them that was OK. I had spent a few days building up trust and gaining a rapport before this. I felt that if K trusted me she would be able to cope better; that was why I explained that her sites would not seem "good" from her point of view but would probably look healthy and good from mine. Gaster (1995) suggests that if the key characteristic in professionals' relations with clients is trust, the key values are integrity and fair conduct. I had not wanted to give K an unrealistic view of what her leg would look like. K was devastated – pavement pizza, raw meat, were adjectives that she used. I spent a long time with her while she cried – looking back grieving for what she had lost. I tried to reiterate that things would improve and that her leg would not look like that forever. Piff (1986) suggests that the reaction that patients receive to their disfigurement strongly influences how they cope in the future. I am pleased that I am aware of this – after 7 years not much of what I see can shock me – but I must help to prepare more junior staff to mask any adverse reactions that they may have.

- How do you think this nurse's use of the literature has helped in her reflection?

'A few days later one of our old patients was re-admitted who had massive skin grafts to his leg that he had received 6 months previously. I asked him if he would mind showing his leg to K, he agreed. K did seem happier knowing that cosmetically the site on her leg would improve. Drench (1994) states that interaction with people who have similar body image deficits but lead active lives seems to help the person make the transition to a new and satisfactory body image. I thought that I was beginning to make headway with K but she remained very emotionally labile – one moment happy the next sobbing uncontrollably. I spent a lot of time with K, listening and talking. I felt that I had built a good trusting relationship at last. Trust according to MacGinley (1993) being very important if a nurse is to help a patient adapt to an altered body image...

'I thought we were doing a good job of promoting acceptance by K of her altered body image, but she was continually very emotional, crying with no seeming end. We tried to get her to see a counsellor to help her psychologically to come to terms with her injury but she would not. I was beginning to get worn out – you can only give so much. When K cried now I found it difficult to empathise. I was beginning to get very judgemental i.e. thinking why doesn't she pull herself together! I haven't got time for this. MacGinley suggests that the nurse should be able to empathise with her patient's feelings e.g. anger depression, in a positive accepting manner without being judgemental. I was no longer able to do this. I found it difficult to care for K. Trying to deal with her strong feeling of despair and anger became difficult and occupied more and more time, until sometimes I left her to cry because it was just too much for me to take. On reflection I should have arranged not to look after her for a few shifts, I should have negotiated a change to give myself a break.'

- How easy is it for a nurse to admit these sorts of feelings?
- How would you feel about sharing similar experiences with a mentor or supervisor?

'Mellor (1996) suggests that getting close to patients can be stressful and lead to burnout. I did not even feel guilty about my actions because all of us as a team of nurses had spent a great deal of time with K. In retrospect looking at the Code of Conduct guidelines (UKCC 1992), especially with respect to clause 5 – "work in an open and co-operative manner with patients, clients and their families, fostering independence and recognise and respect their involvement in planning and delivery of care", we had achieved a high standard of care. Before she was discharged home she was still very emotional and prone to frequent bouts of crying. She had done very well and achieved a great deal: our involving her daily in planning and evaluating her care had helped. Price (1986) advocates the involvement of patients in their care, concluding that they will be more likely to come to terms with their body. K went home and despite the whole team having tried so hard to succeed to the best of our ability – we had failed – no – not failed, just not quite made the grade.

After reflection on this episode, my reading has led me to realise that gaps in our knowledge about normal body image and the stages that a person with altered body image goes through is lacking, in future my care will be enhanced by the knowledge that I have acquired. Price (1990) states that a nurse must become more aware of the normal, as a patient who suffers abrupt body image change may not have had time for that reflection. He has developed a body image model that divides body image into three sections:

(1)   body reality – the way our body is constructed, the way it really is – affected by nature and nurture
(2)   body ideal – how we think we should look
(3)   body presentation – our appearance, dress, jewellery and posture.

He suggests that when one component changes all the components have to adapt. This was difficult for K as so much had changed – her body reality had altered, her ideal had changed as she was dependent and had lost her usual roles and her dress would now change as she felt she should cover her legs. MacGinley (1993) suggests body reality is constantly changing from birth to old age. If K was having the menopause that would indicate yet another change she was enduring. This has sprung to mind as I remembered that she wanted her HRT patches but due to risk of embolism the doctors would not prescribe them. No wonder she had such a hard time, all components were trying to adapt to various changes, some of normal body image and some of altered body image. K had also been quite a plump lady and therefore her skin graft sites appeared very shrunken. Perhaps she had already had negative feelings about her body without adding alterations to it? Salter (1988) suggests people with high self esteem will have a more realistic picture of their body than people with low self esteem. She goes on to say that people with high self esteem will adapt more readily to change in body image. Meisenhelder (1985) defines self esteem as a positive regard for oneself and is a key component in restoring and maintaining mental and physical health. If these concepts had been thought about during K's admission we may have been able to facilitate more acceptance and motivation. Smith (1985) discusses the concept of patient power, the nurse being able to allow the patient to have control over her own destiny. Did we allow this? We did after a stage of complete dependence but we could well have utilised my new knowledge into practice. The answer has to be, yes. By having insight into normal body image for ourselves, as well as K, a more holistic careplan could have been made. I am not saying we did not have a realistic careplan, we did summarise her most specific problems of anxiety, motivation, mobilisation and wound care, but in the light of new knowledge of control, self esteem and how a person adapts to body image it could have been improved.

- Can you identify how the nurse moves around the Gibbs cycle?
- Can you distinguish the levels of reflection (Goodman) that the nurse reaches in her writing?

Exemplar 7

This exemplar was written by a lecturer practitioner taking a post-graduate certificate in education. She is reflecting on her own experiences as a student and concludes by considering how this is useful in her interactions with her own students.

'If I recall when I commenced this course, my motivation was intrinsic. I wanted to learn for learning's sake. I saw a clear relevance of the content matter to what I wanted to do in my current job, as a lecturer practitioner (although there was also some extrinsic motivation, this was not the primary motivation). This relevance and intrinsic motivation are key factors in promoting deep level learning (Marton & Saljo 1976a, 1976b, Fransson 1977, Biggs 1978). I have found it easiest to learn when the topic area had significant relevance and reflected personal interest. For example I am interested in the role of the mentor in supporting students in practice. I wanted to explore this role, in relation to mentors as facilitators of learning, for one of my assignments. I initially felt very enthusiastic, read very widely and felt that I had learnt a lot. I then tried to apply it to the written assignment. I felt confused, disappointed and disillusioned. My biggest disappointment was in myself and in my inability to articulate why I felt the focus that I wanted to explore was appropriate. I started to experience anxiety and my motivation shifted from being intrinsic (an interest in the topic) to needing to do what was required to pass the assignment, an extrinsic motivation (Fransson 1977). This then affected my ability to read, as soon as I adopted a more 'surface' approach (Marton & Saljo 1976a) by not reading for pleasure, but by scanning the literature to find snippets I could use for my assignment. Laurillard (1979) describes how students' approaches to learning change with the task, and are affected by the context of the learning activity. Here, I could clearly see how the task had changed, from being one of relevance and personal interest, to one of completing what was required of me. My anxiety is of great significance here, as I also recognised how my perspective had changed and become less reliable.

My experience of anxiety has been both positive and negative and sometimes both at the same time. The stimulation needed to apply myself to completing course work, has come from my own anxiety of having to meet deadlines. Here, the fear of missing a deadline motivates me to work. Rogers (1986),

Fransson (1977), and Brookfield (1990) recognise that anxiety can be positive and will often act as a motivating force. However, the fear of failure can also act as a block. Getting the balance right between the effects of anxiety is crucial but difficult to achieve as the individual and the environment for learning are affected by many things (Brookfield 1990). Anxiety can be destructive particularly at times of examination or submission of course work, it can impede the individual's ability to concentrate on the task in hand. From my own experience it has felt like a never-ending cycle.'

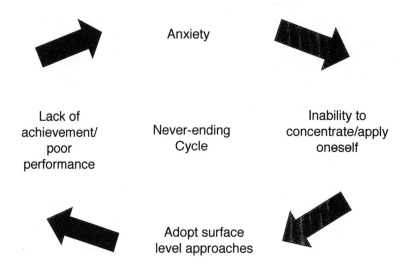

Anxiety

Lack of achievement/ poor performance

Never-ending Cycle

Inability to concentrate/apply oneself

Adopt surface level approaches

Fig. 9.4   The never-ending cycle.

- What do you think of the practitioner's reflective analysis?
- How has the use of the literature helped in this?
- Do you get any feel for the practitioner's sense of self awareness?

'The teacher's role here could be to intervene at any stage of this cycle. Anxiety could be tackled by offering support and positive encouragement. The teacher could help the student with study strategies that promoted better understanding and deeper approaches to learning, such as identifying the relevance of work and by asking pertinent questions. In reflecting on this personal experience I have tried to identify what would have helped me. As a learner, I think it is important to recognise the impact of my own anxiety and to perhaps seek help sooner and be specific in what help I need. As a teacher I need to know the importance of listening to the student and to ask pertinent open questions regarding the difficulties they are experiencing, taking care not to make assumptions. I also believe that when students experience difficulties, it is important not to overwhelm them with new suggestions, and instead spend time making their own ideas work.'

- What stage of the reflective cycle has the practitioner reached?

Exemplar 8

Written by a lecturer practitioner undertaking a Master's programme.

> 'I am attempting to demonstrate the beginning of what Morse (1991) describes as a "connected relationship" and to show the value of "presence" in the caring relationship (Gardener 1985). The extracts from my diary concern a 58-year old man who had suffered a cerebral vascular accident nine months previously during vascular surgery and was left with a dense hemiplegia. He was initially in ICU in a teaching hospital and was now being nursed in a community hospital. This was the first day I nursed him. In any of the types of relationship described by Morse (1991) the crucial point is the interplay between the patient and the nurse.
>
> 'Henry asked me if I lived locally. He made many requests for me to position things around him and on his locker. I complied immediately and with precision. I offered him tea, which he declined, and when I left the room he rang for me shortly afterwards, saying on my return, "I think I'll have that tea after all." I made it just the way he liked it and brought it to him.
>
> 'I recognised this as a test of my dependability, and in wanting to form a relationship with Henry would need to demonstrate this effectively before this could begin. Morse also reports the need for patients to check out about the nurses with other patients.
>
> 'I heard Henry mention my name when talking to the patient in the next bed, perhaps checking out the way I cared for him. Henry asked me all about where I had trained and about my course. When I helped him wash and dress he said positive and affirming things about the thoroughness of my actions and the method I used for his wet shave. I helped him to choose his clothes with some care. I felt him willing to trust me and place himself in my care. I just waited for him to let me in then it all came pouring out.'

- With reference to Johns' structured reflection what are your thoughts about the quality of the practitioner's description of the situation?

> 'I generally found this ward setting to be one where I less often needed to become 'disembodied from the patient" Gadow (1989), she describes this strategy as being used in situations where the nurse has to inflict pain on the patient. This is a common occurrence in acute nursing. The strategy is not only applicable to physical pain but to mental anguish. My awareness of the potential for disembodiment made me use active strategies to stay very much in touch with what Henry wanted to say. There were times when I would have preferred not to have done so. I felt very vulnerable. Retrospectively I think I felt bewilderment, anguish and pain (Gadow).

"The psychiatrist came every day and said cry if you want. When I eventually did I couldn't stop, but they had the windows nailed so you couldn't jump." (Henry's words)

'Gadow explains that the patient's extreme embodiment in their pain, coupled with the nurse's strategy of disembodiment will sever the relationship between the two parties. Much of the literature on the process of inflicting pain in nursing has been built on the basis of torturer and the victim (Daley 1978, Gadow 1989, Laborde 1989). Schroeder (1992) cites Dind (1989) 'Hurting is part of the job" (p. 81).'

'Laborde described common forms of torture as being not very distant from the acts which nurses "routinely perform". There are, however proposed alternatives to these interactions by the promotion of the relationship as all. In this situation the nurse–patient relationship can be negotiated between the nurse and the patient on the basis of the needs of the patient at each encounter (Schroeder). This premise is not valid in the context of the mentally impaired or unconscious patient.

'Henry could recount in graphic detail the misery, powerlessness and intense pain he had endured while supposedly unconscious following his surgery and recovery in the ICU. He spoke of nurses he had a sense of particularly disliking. He was transferred to a medical ward, paralysed, disempowered and depressed. "Can you imagine what it's like? I've shifted 42 tons of sand in a day, then I couldn't even press the call button."

'Henry sounded so angry, he spoke in bursts, blaming the hospital and the surgeon for his situation. I just acknowledged what he had to say, and the pain, and sat and held his hand helping him with a tissue when the tears came. After that we sat in silence and I had a sense of using my presence to calm and comfort him (Gadow 1989, Watson 1985).

'I did a lot of work with Henry and eventually he accepted his situation enough to initiate his choice of placement in a local nursing home. His wife had made it clear that she could not care for him at home and it was a long time before he could accept this.

'I have attempted to demonstrate how descriptive accounts of meaningful experiences, which started life as odd notes in a reflective diary can be analysed and further, that synthesis (new meaning) can be created.'

● What has the practitioner been able to synthesise from her analysis of the situation do you think?

'The piece could have been written without direct reference to the diary extracts but it can be powerful to use the patient's own words and your initial feelings. I have paid some considerable attention to what has been included in this piece to protect the patient's identity and to respect his confidence. It is a very emotional issue for me still because of my deep involvement. The initial subject matter of the reflection does not have to be complex because when you begin to analyse it fully there is so much to consider. I could have continued for several more pages in this example!'

- This exemplar clearly demonstrates the depth of feeling that reflection can unearth for the practitioner and considers the power of sensitive and considerate nursing. What do you think of the points made in this exemplar in relation to your own experiences of practice?
- Consider all the exemplars above and consider where you are able to find evidence of self-awareness, description, critical analysis, synthesis and evaluation. Go back to Sue Atkins' chapter for further information on these 'building blocks' for reflection.

Conclusion

I have deliberately chosen exemplars from a range of practitioners with varied experiences and educational preparation. They demonstrate differing ability as the nurse gains in experience, knowledge and skills. Of course this may not be the case for every practitioner since it depends on how experience, knowledge and skills are utilised. It is worth noting that the personal styles of reflective writing are undoubtedly varied. It appears to me that the development of the 'building blocks' of reflection, that is self awareness, description, analysis, synthesis and evaluation are essential in order to facilitate a growth in reflective ability.

The exemplars are powerful, particularly in their ability to highlight analytical thinking about practice and a willingness and ability to change and be open-minded. They provide narrative evidence that nurses can and do use the power of storytelling to unearth what nursing is about. These exemplars also demonstrate to me that reflection can be painful, although such an outlet for the exploration of feelings can be cathartic for the practitioner. Finally, these exemplars show the potential of reflective practitioners in their ability to examine and act upon the actual realities of practice and to learn from experience.

Now is your chance to try it.

References

Biggs, J.B. (1978) Individual and group differences in study processes. *British Journal of Educational Psychology*, **48**, pp266 –279.

Boud, D., Keogh, R. & Walker, D (1985) (eds) *Reflection: Turning experience into learning*, Kogan Page, London.

Brookfield, S. (1990) *The Skilful Teacher. On technique, trust and responsiveness in the classroom*, Jossey-Bass Inc, San Francisco.

Burnard, P. (1991) Improving through reflection. *Journal of District Nursing*, May 10–12.

Carr, E.C.J. (1996) Reflecting on clinical practice: hectoring talk or reality. *Journal of Clinical Nursing*, **5**, 289–95.

Cronan, L. (1993) Management of the patient with altered body image. *British Journal of Nursing* **2**(5), 257–61.

Cullingford, S. (1991) Learning from experience. *Senior Nurse.* **11** (6) Nov/Dec, 25–28.

Daley, M. (1978) *Gyn/Ecology: The meta-ethics of radical feminism,* Beacon Press, Boston.

Dewing, J. (1989) Altered body image. *Surgical Nurse,* **2** (4), 17–20.

Dind, C. (1989) Teaching nurses about torture. *International Nursing Review,* **36** (3), 81–2.

Drench, M. (1994) Changes in body image secondary to disease. *Rehabilitation Nursing,* **19** (1) 31–6.

Driscoll, J. (1994) Reflective practice for practise. *Senior Nurse,* **13** (7), Jan/Feb.

Fransson, A. (1977) On qualitative differences in learning IV, Effects of intrinsic motivation and extrinsic test anxiety on processes and outcome. *British Journal of Educational Psychology,* **47**, 244–57.

French, H.P. (1979) Reassurance: a nursing skill? *Journal of Advanced Nursing,* **4**, 627–34.

Gadow, S. (1989) Clinical subjectivity: advocacy in silent patients. *Nursing Clinics of North America,* **24** (12), 535–41.

Gardener, D. (1985) Presence In Bulecheck, McClosky and Aydelotte (eds) *Nursing Interventions – Treatments for Nursing Diagnosis,* WB Saunders, Philadelphia.

Gaster, L. (1995) *Quality in Public Services. Managers Choice,* Open University Press, Buckingham.

Gibbs, G. (1988) *Learning by Doing. A guide to teaching and learning methods,* Further Education Unit, Oxford Polytechnic (*now* Oxford Brookes University), Oxford.

Goodman, J. (1984) Reflection and teacher education: a case study and theoretical analysis. *Interchange,* **15** (3), 9–26.

Hargreaves, J. (1997) Using patients: exploring the ethical dimension of reflective practice in nurse education. *Journal of Advanced Nursing,* **25**, 223–8.

Heinrich, K.T. (1992) The intimate dialogue: journal writing by students. *Nurse Educator,* **17**, Nov/Dec, 17–23.

James, C.R. & Clarke, B.A. (1994) Reflective practice in nursing: issues and implications for nursing education. *Nurse Education Today,* **14**, 82–90.

Jarvis, P. (1992) Reflective practice and nursing. *Nurse Education Today,* **12**, 174–81.

Jones, R.K. & Jones, P.A. (1975) *Sociology in Medicine,* EUP, London.

Johns, C. (1993) Professional supervision. *Journal of Nursing Management,* **1**, 9–18.

Johns, C. (1994) Guided reflection. In Palmer, A., Burns, S. & Bulman, C. (eds) *Reflective Practice in Nursing. The Growth of the Professional Practitioner,* Blackwell Science Oxford.

Johns, C. (1995a) The value of reflective practice for nursing. *Journal of Clinical Nursing,* **4**, 23–30.

Johns, C. (1995b) Framing learning through reflection within Carper's fundamental ways of knowing in nursing. *Journal of Advanced Nursing*, **22**, 226–34.

Laborde, J. (1989) Torture: A nursing concern. *Image*, **21** (1), 31–3.

La Puma, J., Schiedemayer, D.L., Guyas, A.E. Siegler, M. (1988) Talking to comatose patients. *Archives of Neurology*, **45** January, 20–22.

Laurillard, D. (1979) The processes of student learning. *Higher Education*, **8**, 395–409.

Lindsay, K.W., Bone, I. & Callander, R. (1991) *Neurology and Neurosurgery Illustrated*, Churchill Livingstone, London.

MacGinley, K.J. (1993) Nursing care of the patient with altered body image. *British Journal of Nursing*, **2** (22), 1098–1102.

Marton, F. & Saljo, R. (1976a) On qualitative differences in learning 1. Outcome and process. *British Journal of Educational Psychology*, **46**, 4–11.

Marton, F. & Saljo, R. (1976b) On qualitative differences in learning 2. Outcome as a function of the learner's conception of the task. *British Journal of Educational Psychology*, **46**, 186–192.

Meisenhelder, J. (1985) Self-esteem; A closer look at clinical interventions. *International Journal of Nursing Studies*, **22** (2), 127–35.

Mellor, D. (1996) Altered body image. *Professional Nurse*, **11** (5), 296–8.

Mezirow, J. (1981) A critical theory of adult learning and education. *Adult Education*, **32**, 3–24.

Morse, J. (1991) Negotiating commitment and involvement in the nurse patient relationship. *Journal of Advanced Nursing*, **16**, 455–68.

Newell, R. (1992) Anxiety, accuracy and reflection: the limits of professional development. *Journal of Advanced Nursing*, **17**, 1326–33.

Paterson, B.L. (1995) Developing and maintaining reflection in clinical journals. *Nurse Education Today*, **15**, 211–20.

Piff, C. (1986) Facing up to disfigurement. *Nursing Times*, **82**, 16–17.

Powell, T. (1994) *Head Injury: A Practical Guide*, Oxon, Winslow Press Limited.

Price, B. (1986) Keeping up appearances. *Nursing Times*, **82** (37), 58–61.

Price, B. (1990) *Body Image: Nursing concepts and care*, Prentice Hall, London.

Richardson, G. & Maltby, H. (1995) Reflection on practice: enhancing student learning. *Journal of Advanced Nursing*, **22**, 235–42.

Rogers, A. (1986) *Teaching Adults*, Open University Press, Buckingham.

Salter, M. (1988) *Altered Body Image: The Nurse's Role*, John Wiley and Sons, Chichester.

Saylor, C.R. (1990) Reflection and professional education: art, science and competency. *Nurse Education*, **15** (2) March/April, 8–11.

Schön, D. (1983) *The Reflective Practitioner*, Basic Books, New York.

Schroeder, C. (1992) The process of inflicting pain in nursing. In Gaut, D. A. (ed) *The Presence of Caring in Nursing*, National League for Nursing, New York.

Shields, E. (1995) Reflection and learning in student nurses. *Nurse Education Today*, **15**, 452–8.

Smith, F.B. (1985) Patient Power. *American Journal of Nursing*, Nov. 1260–62.

Stephenson, S. (1994) Reflection–A Student's Perspective. In Palmer, A., Burns, S. & Bulman, C. (eds) *Reflective Practice in Nursing. The Growth of the Professional Practitioner*. Blackwell Science, Oxford.

Street, A. (1991) *From Image to Action: Reflection in nursing practice*. Deakin University Press, Geelong.

Taylor, S. & Field, D. (1993) *Sociology of Health and Health Care*, Blackwell Science, Oxford.

UKCC (1992) *The Scope of Professional Practice*. UKCC, London.

Watson, J. (1985) *Nursing: Human Science and Human Care. A theory of nursing*, Appleton-Century-Crofts, Connecticut.

Wellard, S.J. & Bethune, E. (1996) Reflective journal writing in nurse education: whose interests does it serve? *Journal of Advanced Nursing*, **24**, 1077–82.

Wright, B.A. (1982) Value laden beliefs and principles of rehabilitation. *Rehabilitation Nursing*, 34–6.

Wright, B. (1986) *Caring in Crisis*. Churchill Livingstone, London.

My thanks to the following people for their contributions to the chapter and their willingness to share their reflective work with others: Elizabeth Austin, Melanie Batt, Nicki Bower, Kerry Davidson, Nadine Jackson, Pam Sharp.

Index